Pushing the

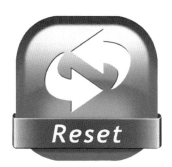

Button

The busy professional's guide to
a healthy lifestyle you will love

Linda Orr Easthouse

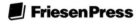 **FriesenPress**

Suite 300 – 990 Fort Street
Victoria, BC, Canada V8V 3K2
www.friesenpress.com

Copyright © 2014 by Linda Orr Easthouse
First Edition — 2014

ISBN
978-1-4602-5661-9 (Hardcover)
978-1-4602-5662-6 (Paperback)
978-1-4602-5663-3 (eBook)

1. Health & Fitness, General

Distributed to the trade by The Ingram Book Company

TABLE OF CONTENTS

Dedication

To my family:
Randy, Greg, and Tim

Without your love and support, I would never have learned what I now know or become what I am. Thank you.

Following this plan will help me be there for you for many years more. 60 is just starting middle age!

To my teachers, students, and clients:

I learn so much each time we interact. The opportunity to sort out an energy field, to listen to what the body on my table wants to say, to be the interpreter of what shows up is such a gift from each of you. Thank you.

Special thanks to Jimmy Scott for the wealth of Health Kinesiology you share with the world. Much appreciation to Vivian Klein and Sandra Gust, wonderful instructors who shared their knowledge, talents, and gifts with me and all their students; and who act as mentors and guides along the way.

Praise for
Pushing the Reset Button

As a person who has led an extremely busy and hectic lifestyle, I pulled out all the stops physically and mentally to keep the adrenal rush going to maintain my pace. As a result, approximately one year ago I suffered complete burn out and became extremely ill. I had seen numerous doctors, here in Canada and the U.S., who could only get my health improving marginally before I would start relapsing. Nothing seemed to be working. Due to the urging of a loving friend, I was referred to Linda and made an appointment to see her almost immediately. I was at my wits end and being chronically ill for so long was taking a heavy toll. Since seeing her approximately two months ago now, my health has improved dramatically in all aspects more than I could have ever expected in such a short period of time. Linda's methods of healing and improving health (regardless of your current status) are very logical and extraordinary aspects of which are described in this book. Understanding that not everyone is fortunate enough to seek assistance from her one-on-one, this book is phenomenal in outlining the healing protocols that can be used at your own pace to gain optimal health, mind and body. I plan on using Linda's healing methods not only until

I achieve full recovery with her, but for the rest of my life to maintain optimal health."

S. Khan,
Calgary, Alberta, Canada

Pushing the

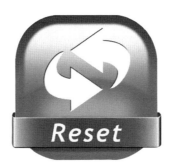

Button

The busy professional's guide to
a healthy lifestyle you will love

Introduction:
Jimmy Scott, PhD

Many years ago I used to do a lecture called "How to be healthy even though you smoke, drink, take drugs, eat junk food, and live riotously". It was a popular lecture and I soon discovered that most people want to do all those things and also be healthy without any other special effort. What I discussed in the lecture was that the more bad things you do to your health, the more good things you must do to counterbalance that. The sneaky part is that when you start doing those good things you automatically start losing your craving for the bad things. In those days there was no "reset button".

Many people know, for example, that to stop smoking is very difficult. What I found with smokers was that if we work on improving their good habits after a while they lose their craving for smoking without us having to deal with it specifically. In other words we often achieved great success just by having people do the right things for themselves without focusing on the bad habits. On the other hand, these days we do have some very powerful techniques to reduce stress in a person's life and to make it easier for them to change their habits. This book is a wonderful guide to much of that process. By stretching out that change process over several months people are more likely to follow the program than if we just "push" them to change all at once. Linda Orr Easthouse has provided a good blueprint and many helpful tools for people wanting to change their lives and enjoy that process. The old "no gain without pain" is obsolete. Using the right techniques and modern information people can painlessly change their lives in ways they would never have imagined previously. In doing so they often do not even realize that they pushed their "reset button". If you want a better healthier life then follow the program in this book, and you will like the results.

Jimmy Scott, PhD
Founder, Health Kinesiology/Natural Bioenergetics

How to read this book

Welcome to the rest of your life.

This is a step-by-step guide to get you where you want to be.

To change your life there are five strands or aspects you need to give attention to on a daily basis. Doing a little bit of each one every day will turn your life around. So the five strands I focus on are:

1.   Retrain your thinking –read and reflect for 10 minutes

2.   Redefine your diet –read 10 minutes and choose new food habits

3.   Reduce stress –meditations, breathing, and relaxation for 15 minutes

4.   Restart your exercise –just do it for 20 minutes

5.   Reduce the toxins –read 10 minutes and clean out the chemicals from your home

With just five 10-20 minute chunks in your day you can create serious change.

If you're like me, a plan like this can be a little daunting. So… breathe, relax, and dive in. I've tried to set it up in a way that regardless of who you are, your personality and your style, you will benefit from this guide. If you're one of those who likes to just jump in with both feet and get the pain over with, then do all five strands at the same time. Go for it. Thirty days from now you'll feel awesome. Along the way you're going to learn a lot, try a lot, and change a lot. But you'll get a lot done. You will be on your way to a long and healthy life.

On the other hand, if you're a little bit more like me, and you read the whole book through and then say to yourself, "This is overwhelming," or, "I don't know that I can do this," what I suggest is approaching the plan by doing part of it for the first pass and then go back each month and add other strands as you build it up.

Whatever way works for you, works! It does not matter. If it takes you a year to get through all five strands and build that routine, that's great. If you do it in 30 days, that's great too. Do what works for you – just keep doing it. One day at a time, one change at a time. Keep building them up; pretty soon it will be a whole new routine, a whole new lifestyle and you will kick-start your life to be where you really want to be.

My Story

I've been where you are. I am a busy professional mother. I run my own business and I have done so for 10 years. I was a busy professional working in a non-profit for 18 years prior to that. During that time we raised two boys. Both of them had a lot of medical and learning issues. They are wonderful, warm, gifted dyslexics with very high IQs but had a hard time putting anything on paper or keeping their attention on only one thing for long periods of time. You can guess what some of those challenges were like. During this time, it was quite easy to lose myself, to find that I was spending all of my time looking after other people, doing things for other people, just keeping all the balls in the air, running from crisis to crisis. I lost my center. I lost my space.

When that happens, when you lose yourself, at some point, you have to come up for a breather or face a total crash with a meltdown. Maybe the kids have gotten older, maybe you've changed jobs like I did, or maybe you've done something to create a new space. Good for you.

If you haven't yet, now is the time to do that. That new space can be just a decision to look after yourself. It can be the choice to recognize it is time for your needs to be a part of the equation. It is time to care for the caregiver, or the caregiver will soon burn out. Or maybe you've already reached burnout and you need to rebuild. Either way, this is a plan to help you get there.

MAY I TELL YOU SOME OF MY STORY?

My journey in Health Kinesiology began in 2002. We had just moved to Canada from Peru. Both my children had suffered from chronic allergies to foods, pollens, molds, dusts, everything! They had developed asthma, and had endured ear/nose/throat infections for many years. An acquaintance at work offered to have a look at them after he heard they had been in emergency again, over the cottonwood trees. He said he did "a little natural health therapy", just as a ministry to help people.

We had already done all the diets, acupuncture, nutritional supplements and everything else we knew, but both kids were on two kinds of puffers and two antihistamines. It seemed so deceptively simple. Just a couple of sessions and they started getting better. Three months later, they were off the puffers. Six months later they were off the antihistamines. Allergies no longer control their lives.

About three months in, I asked him to have a look at my allergies. I just had a few but wanted to feel what was happening and learn more about it. At the end of the session, he said, "By the way your thyroid isn't working." I knew that, it had never worked. I had been on meds my whole life. He asked if I wanted it fixed! When I told him that Doctors had always told me it wasn't fixable, he replied, "We can see what your body wants to do with it." Two sessions later, my thyroid clicked on like a switch and I was able to go off my meds. My blood tests are still perfect—better than they were on the meds.

At that point I was hooked. I asked him to teach me what he did. Of course, he said no but that I should go take one of the training courses. So in early 2003 I flew to the US and later to the UK and started the road to becoming a fully certified practitioner of Health Kinesiology. It has been a long but satisfying journey. My job as a therapist is the most fulfilling, satisfying work I have ever done. Helping others be the best they can be physically, emotionally, mentally and spiritually gives me purpose to keep pursuing higher training and greater experience that will make me a better practitioner and better person. I want to share as much as I can with you here. Of course you might need some of the therapy too but starting with what you can do for yourself is a great launching pad.

This is not a research book. This is not going to give you all the scientific studies and convince you of why you need to do all this stuff. You may have already done that research, or you may be just starting the journey and want the list of what you need to do. It can be overwhelming. There is so much information out there and it is just more than you have time to sort out. This book sorts it out for you. The whole purpose here is to lay out a plan that you can do step by step, choosing as many strands at a time as you feel comfortable with. If right now you're in "overwhelm" mode, and all you can do is one strand at a time, then do one strand at a time. Every little step moves you one step closer to getting your life back on track.

This was my plan. This is what got me from stressed out, close to burnout, thyroid not functioning, foggy, frightened about how to move forward, and frustrated, to living life on my terms and enjoying my life and my family again. No, life is not perfect, my kids as young adults still have issues, but I handle it differently. I don't stress myself out. I can keep my center. I have my priorities in place no matter what happens.

This isn't about a quick fix or a magic bullet. This isn't about a diet that will get you an instant weight loss, or a "Get Fit Quick" program. This is about creating, crafting and designing a lifestyle that you can live with for the rest of your life: One that will set a solid foundation for you to move forward into good health, into a solid, clean, healthy lifestyle that you can maintain. I don't want you to just hold your breath and get it over with. I want you to invest your time and energy into something that makes sense and creates a solid foundation from which you can make decisions on a daily basis of what you will do and what you won't do, how you're going to do it and how you're not going to do it.

There is a lot of wisdom in the old illustration, "Take a big jar and fill it with sand, gravel and rocks. If you put the sand in the bottom first, and then the gravel, there's no room for the big rocks. But if you put the big rocks in first, then you pour the gravel around it, then you put the sand in then you can even pour some water in. You can get twice as much in, because the priorities are there first." These strands are like the big rocks. These set the foundation for you. When you get this part of your lifestyle down, the rest of it will fill in around the pieces, allowing you to do what you need to do, giving you your flexibility and allowing you to move you forward in a healthy lifestyle no matter what life throws at you.

The Plan

Put on your running shoes, and let's go

A little bit about how we're going to deal with this. I have divided the month into five weeks – four complete weeks and the fifth week is just the last three days of the month.

Week 1 – We are focusing on "**I know who I am, and I am OK.**" Most of us, by the time we are ready to read this book, well, we don't feel OK, and we're not sure who "me" is anymore. For a week we're going to take some time and we're really going to focus on "Who am I, and it is okay whoever I am." To do that, we are going to introduce Meridian tracing, which is an energy exercise to help refocus and center the body and mind. We are going to look at some quick ways to move your body's dietary needs in a different direction, and help you get some process into your daily routine. We are going to start with very gentle exercises – just walking for 20 minutes a day – and begin to clean out garbage. Rejecting toxins is a huge part of getting your life under control; so much of the tiredness and the lethargy and chronic not feeling well comes from the garbage in our environment. So we'll take a look at that.

Week 2 – We are going to focus on the future, and really get it into our heads that "I create my own future, I am the master of my ship, I am the creator of my life; my lifestyle is what I make it to be." Mentally, there are things we can do to control that. We'll have a look at some of those. How do we create our future? Why do we do it? What do we do to change the way our future is headed now? I'm going to teach you some meditation techniques, and give you a few fun exercises to do there. The first major diet change is to reduce the wheat in your diet; I know that sounds awful, but it is important, and we'll talk about why. We are going to add a little bit of yoga to your walking routine, just to give variety, and get some stretching going on as well, nothing serious, just enough to get your body into a different flexibility mode. Rejecting toxins: we are going to look at all the body products you use and what is wrong with them, what you can do to change that, and why you need to change that. There is a lot of research out there, lots of books. I will recommend some resources for you to read, and I will give you some very basic steps for cleaning up your body products.

Week 3 – I am what I eat. This week we're really focusing on the eating aspect of things. What you think determines what you eat. I know that's hard to believe, but it's true. What you think determines what you eat. For reducing stress, we'll look at some breathing exercises; there are a lot of fun things you can do for that. In refining your diet, we are going to tackle that sugar monster. For exercise, we are going to teach you the Tibetan 5 Exercise, to give you a little variety just in case you were getting bored with yoga and walking by now. On rejecting toxins, we're going to look at the GMO issue and why and how those are so bad for you, as well as what you can do to avoid them and get them out of your diet.

Week 4 – By now you have probably hit the self-sabotage button. Most of us do. Week 4 is all about "I can stop self-sabotage." There are ways around it. I'm going to teach you some exercises called the "Emotional Stress Release" and the "BS Eliminator" to help you reduce your stress and get yourself back on track. We are going to remove dairy from your diet; I know that sounds scary but it's really not. There are lots of great alternatives out there, and there are lots of reasons why you don't want to drink it or eat it. With exercise, we are going to add one day of high-intensity training. The rest of the week is carrying on your yoga and walking, or Tibetan 5s, whichever you prefer, and then that one day of intensity training. You only need one day a week, and less than 30 minutes to get your desired results. On the toxin issue, we're going to go with hormones and antibiotics. There are hidden sources of both of those that you probably don't even know you're getting, but they're affecting you and your family and you need to get them out.

Week 5: The last few days… a short week. I know it's hard to believe that we've made it this far. We're focusing on "I become what I believe I am." Let that sink in for a little bit. For stress, we're going to talk about rest and sleep. For refining your diet, we're going to talk about fats, the good ones and the bad ones. With exercise, you are just going to keep going with the same things you've been doing. You've got a good routine up, now it is just maintaining. And for toxins, we're going to talk about things like using plastics and all those nasties that we take for granted in our society and our houses, and we have no idea what they are doing to us. Well, we do have some ideas of what they are doing to us and want to get them out of our houses.

Doesn't sound too bad, does it? You can do that for 30 days. Once you've done it for 30 days, then it is just a matter of repeating, refining, picking up nuances on it, recognizing new sources of things that we thought we had gotten rid of, finding better ways to replace it, and building until it just becomes a natural routine that this is the way we live. When you live this way, you'll be happier, you'll be healthier, you'll have more energy, and you will have control back in your life. Yes, you'll still be a busy professional; yes, there will still be days where things go out the window, but you will have the bedrock to work up from. You will have the routine down that works for you. You can come back and repeat the 30-day workout whenever you want, or you can just plod away, applying these principles throughout the rest of your life to maintain a long, healthy, happy life.

Looking forward to meeting with you. Give me a shout on Facebook www.facebook.com/easthousehealth or follow me on my blog on the website www.easthousecentre.com. Check out my free gift for you at www.lindaeasthouse.com

> Love to talk to you,
> Linda Orr Easthouse

Week 1:
I know who I am, and I am OK

Living in the present, doing the best you can with what you have, accepting that for the moment you are where you are and it's OK.

~ Linda Orr Easthouse

This first week is all about, "**I know who I am and I am OK.**" It's about figuring out who "me" is now that you're caught in a whirlwind of family, business, life and work, all of those things that have taken you away from your center. Or maybe you never really found your center? This week you're going to spend some time figuring out who "me" is, who you really want to be, and realizing that no matter where you are, you're OK. It is OK to start from wherever you're at, and every step you take will take you closer to where you want to be. It's a journey. It is not a race. One step at a time. One change at a time. And it's OK if you miss a day. It's OK if you screw up a day. It's OK if you don't do something you're supposed to do. Every step forward moves you a step closer, and even if you take a step backwards you can always take another step forwards. Give yourself grace, and accept that where you are is where you are. No blame or scapegoat needed. Just set your compass for somewhere else and start moving.

It is OK if you're starting from, "I'm completely stressed out," or "I'm overweight," or "I have too many things to do," or even "I can't even think about me, I have way more critical issues on my hands." That's a good place to start from. Every little step you take away from that will help you find your center, and get you back to being you. Let's jump into the journey, and go from here.

<hr/>

DAY 1

If someone wishes for good health, one must first ask oneself if he, or she, is ready to do away with the reasons for his illness. Only then is it possible to help him.

~ Hippocrates

Retrain your thoughts.

I have often found myself wishing for good health and then realizing I wasn't ready to give up the daily things I do that were contributing to not having good health. Hippocrates' wisdom helps us realize that it's only when we're ready to deal with the causes that we can get rid of the symptoms. The causes are the things we do every day: the things we put in our mouth, the things we don't do in terms of exercise, the choices we make at the grocery store, the choice we make to worry and to allow stress to set off that chemical flood through the body. When I'm ready to make changes to what I do on a daily basis, then I can begin to fulfil my wish for good health.

So take a moment and jot down here some of the habits that you need to change that will help you move forward on your road to good health. What are some of the daily choices you make that you can change? The reasons for your illness are found in your daily habits. When you're ready to face the reasons, when you're ready to change the habits, then you can address the illness. This guide will help you.

My reasons for not being healthy in mind, body, and spirit:

1. _____

2. _____

3. _____

4. _____

5. _____

Reduce your stress

I'll bet if you're like me, one of the things you jotted down there was you need to reduce your stress. You need to lower your stress levels. This week we're going to teach you a little exercise that will help you to do that. I will break you in easy. We will do a simple de-stressing activity that you can do daily for the rest of the month, the rest of the year, or the rest of your life, that will always help you to get centered and grounded and bring your energy back into a more focused and smooth flow. There will just be the one thing to learn for this week and you'll do the same thing every day this week. It's called Meridian Tracing.

I'm going to give you a website where you can go and watch a video to follow along if you'd like – go to www.easthouse-centre.com, choose the Resources page, choose the Self-Help videos and look for Meridian tracing. What you find there on the video is the point-by-point exact flow of the meridians. You don't need to be that specific; we do what we call the "quick type." The quick Meridian tracing is based on the understanding that energy follows intention. Your body knows where your meridians are, and if you intend to follow the meridians, even if you don't cover every little zigzag that's on the video, your body will run the energy down that meridian. I'm going to walk you through it, and it's very easy to do.

Take your hands and hold them about 2–3 inches out from your body. Use your fingers as pointers all together, very relaxed. You need to be standing, and start with your fingers under your eyes on your cheekbones. You are simply going to run your hands 2–3 inches away from your body all the way down the front of your legs to your toes, out to the ends of your toes and back up the way you came, until you get just above the breasts. Then go out like a candy cane to the sides of the chest just underneath the armpits, about four inches down right on the bra line for women, doing both hands at the same time. For those of you who are curious, those are the stomach and spleen meridians. Let's do that one again just so that you get the idea.

Start underneath the eyes, all the way down to the toes, back up to just above the breast and out in an arc like a candy cane, to the sides of the body about 4 inches below the armpits.

Now take your left hand and hold it out. Take your right hand, start at your left armpit and sweep underneath your arm all the way out to the fingertips, around the ends of the fingers and back up across the top of your arm, over your shoulder and up to the side of your face. Repeat the other side; hold your right arm out. Start with the left hand at the armpit and run underneath the arm, out over the ends of the fingers and back across the top of the hand, over the arm to the shoulders, and up to the right side of your face.

Now let's start between your eyebrows. One hand on each side, sweep up over the top of your head, and down past your neck as far as you can reach. Bring your arms around the other side and reach back up as far as you can go. Yes, there will be a gap but that's OK; the body knows that's where the energy needs to go. Continue to trace down the middle of your back, down through your hips, down through the back of the glutes (buttocks). Down behind the knees to the sides of the legs, all the way down to your little toe, and then bring your hands around and go underneath your foot to the ball of your foot, and bring your hands back up coming in the insides of your legs, up through the groin area between the breasts, right up to your collar bone.

Then you're going to do your arms again the exact same way you did it last time on both sides.

Take your left arm and hold it out. Take your right hand, start at your armpit and sweep under your left arm all the way out to the fingers, around the ends of the fingers and back up across the top of your arm, over your shoulder and up to the side of your face. Repeat the other side; hold your right hand out. Start with the left hand at the armpit and run underneath the arm, out over the ends of the fingers and back across the top of the hand, over the arm to the shoulders to the right side of your face.

This third one, we're going to do from the sides of your eyes. Go down the sides of your face to your shoulder to the sides of your torso. Down the side of your torso, down the side of your hips to the outside of your knees all the way down to the outside of the foot. Come across the front of the toes to the big toe, and straight up the front of the legs up just inside the ball of the ankle, just on the inside of the kneecap and stop on your ribcage under the breasts between rib 7 and rib 8.

Again, repeat the arms on both sides.

Then we're going to close it with the Zipper. One hand in front of the pubic bone, one hand behind at the sacroiliac (tailbone), and you're simply going to draw them both up together till you get to the neck. Then, the front one is going to stop underneath the bottom lip and the back one is going to continue up over the top of the head down the ridge of the nose and stop above the top lip. Pull your hands away from the center line, because you don't want to unzip what you just zipped up, and go back and do it again. Pubic bone front and tailbone back, straight up the middle, front stops at bottom of lips and back goes all the way around to the top of the lips. Separate your hands out again and do it one more time.

That's Meridian tracing. You're going to do that three times. So, you've already been through the entire process once; go back and do it again, then do it a third time. I know it seems like a lot at this point, but it's really simple once you've done it every day of the week. You'll have it memorized and you won't even have to look at the papers.

What you need to remember is you go down the front, back up the front to the sides of the arms, underneath from the armpit over the ends of the fingers, back up the top to the side of the face on both arms, starting at the eyebrows over the head down the back, up the front and then do the arms again, starting at the sides of the eyes down the outside of the body, up the inside of the legs and torso to the ribs, do the arms again, and zip three times.

You'll find that after you've done this, you'll feel calmer, more energetic, and warmer. Pay attention to how you feel before and how you feel afterwards. What it's doing is getting your energy flowing and smoothing out the flow, helping it open up blockages, helping it get through tight places, helping it calm down places where it's running too fast.

Reducing your stress is as simply as getting your energy flowing smoothly. For this week, do it every day. Build a habit and do it for a whole month; you'll be glad you did.

Redefine your diet

For this week we're focusing on water and juice. Many of you don't really like to drink a lot of water. I want to spend some time discussing why water is important. Water is the fluid in your brain that allows neurons to send signals from one dendrite to another. Your brain functions in a salty solution of water, basically. When there isn't enough water in the brain and the brain gets dehydrated, those messages don't jump as well. You all know that water is an ideal way to spread electric shock. In a flood, electricity always gets turned off first because if you step in the water and the water is in contact with the electrical socket, you will get electrocuted. Well, your brain requires that electric circuit in order to pass its messages from one brain cell to the next. When there isn't enough water in the brain, you don't get messages. You get confusion, you get "slow thinking," and you get fogginess. This is often a problem with elderly – their thinking is slow, confused, and foggy because they're not drinking enough water, in part because they don't want to get up and go pee in the middle of the night. Because they are having urinary issues, they lower their water, hoping to solve one problem but creating another.

By the time you feel thirsty, it's way too late. Thirst is the last signal you get that your brain is low on water. By the time you feel thirsty, your brain is already dehydrated. So, how much water do you need? For most people it's 2–3L per day. For those of you in the United States, it's 2–3 quarts per day. The most important point is that the water must be clean, purified water. Water that comes from your tap has chemicals in it. Water that comes from your tap has hormones in it, because all those people that take medications, drugs, hormone replacement therapy, etc. pee it into the waste water. The waste water gets cleaned; however, those very fine tiny molecules get through the system and end up back in the rivers and in the next town downstream. The river is coming in with those chemicals; those hormones are in the "clean" water. So, get yourself a good filter. And no, Brita doesn't count. Get a real filter that will take out contaminants down to very fine microns. It doesn't have to be very expensive; the one I personally use is called *Aquasana*. There are many good ones out there. There's lots of research out there, you can do your own, but make sure you're getting one that gets those hormones out.

The other major thing that you need to be sure is **not** in your water is fluoride. Fluoride is a neurotoxin. Fluoride is a waste product from the aluminum smelting industry. They get rid of their toxic waste by selling it to cities to put it in water so that they don't have to dispose of it. Fluoride does not belong in our drinking water. It has been proven to lower IQ, and has been proven to make populations more docile and compliant. So get the fluoride out of your water. Doesn't matter how you do it, just get it out.

If you choose to use reverse osmosis water, make sure that you are adding the proper minerals back in. Plants, animals and people who use reverse osmosis water REQUIRE natural minerals to be returned to the water because it takes out everything. Yes, you get completely clean water, but on the other hand, you lose the natural minerals that you're supposed to be getting. The best way to get them back in is to ensure that you're eating fresh green vegetables and using natural pink sea salt. The pink sea salt is higher in minerals than the white sea salt; therefore, if you're using reverse osmosis then you need to be using the pink sea salt, which gets you a broader spectrum of the minerals than you would get with just the regular sea salt. So, pure water, lots of it, replaces the other things you're drinking. Obviously if you're drinking 2–3 liters of pure water a day, you don't need to be drinking pop or soda or sugary juices or coffee or tea with sugar in it. Replace your liquids with water. For starters, it's cheaper, way better for you, and feeds your brain. Get water in your diet.

Restart your exercise

For this week we're starting with the very basics. Carve out 20 minutes and go out for a walk – a good brisk walk. If your weather permits, do it outside, unless you're in a highly polluted city environment, in which case you maybe want to do it inside where there is a little more air control and filtering. If at all possible, get outside. Just 20 minutes and walk. I don't care where you walk or how fast you walk, just go and do it. Twenty minutes won't kill you. You can do it on your lunch hour, or you can do it in the evening – after dinner is a great time. Just get out and walk, and I know how hard that can be, but do it.

Rejecting toxins

This week we're focusing on the household cleaners that you can use. Why is that so important? Some of the most toxic things that you come into contact with that create significant stress on your liver and on your kidneys are the things that you use to clean your house. Check and see how many products you have in your house that say "antibacterial." Every antibacterial product that is in your house needs to be thrown out. The antibacterial products all have Triclosan in them. Triclosan is one of the hormone-disrupting chemicals that severely affect you and the environment. Every time you wash your hands with that stuff it goes down the drain and into our sewers and causes problems to all the aquatic life. Fish, frogs, birds that bathe in them and eat plants that suck it up – they are all getting an overload of estrogen from that stuff and it is creating havoc in their environments as well.

The crazy thing is that that antibacterial soap doesn't actually kill bacteria unless it's been in contact with it for 10 minutes. How can you even wash your hands for 10 minutes? I don't. It's just a sales and marketing pitch. Pure old regular soap will do just as good a job and not pollute the environment, and not put extra estrogen hormones into your nice, wet skin that absorbs everything right in. So, for today's toxin to remove, get rid of the antibacterial toxins. Whether that is hand soap, dishwashing soap, wipe-up cloths or hand sanitizer, read the labels. If it says Triclosan, don't use it. Don't forget to check your toothpaste. Colgate total also contains it.

DAY 2

Trade your Expectation for Appreciation and the world changes instantly.

~ Tony Robbins

Retrain your thoughts:

It's all about perspective, isn't it? If you expect that this is going to be really hard and that there will be a hundred interruptions and things that need your attention, then that is what you will find. However, if you just shift your focus a little and appreciate, think, "I have a plan, someone has done the hard work to figure it out, all I have to do is take this baby step," your attitude changes your behaviour.

You can do five minutes here, come back after that interruption and do 10 minutes, and over the day you look back and it will be done. Look around and be grateful for having a house with enough room that you can stand up and do your Meridian tracing.

Be grateful you have a computer or an iPad to read on, or a book in your hands. Think of this as a recipe for the rest of your life. The more times you make the same recipe, the easier it gets, until you don't even need the book, you just do it. Your expectation can be useful. You expect that the recipe is going to work, and it helps you trust the process and do all the steps. That positive expectation is really an appreciation of the work that has gone into the recipe you are following.

Our expectations can get us into a lot of trouble, or our appreciation can get us a lot of peace and cooperation.

Reduce your stress:

Time to do your Meridian tracing again.

Stand up. Hands under the eyes, down to the toes, back up in a candy cane arch to the sides of the body. Armpits, under the arm, over the hand, back up across the top of the shoulder and onto the side of the face.

Hands between the eyebrows, up and over the head, reach around and continue on down the back to the sides of the foot. Starting under the inside of the foot, go up behind the ankle ball, up the inside of the legs over the groin, up to the collarbone. Do the arms again.

Start beside the eyes, going down the outside of the torso, down the outside of the legs, to the toes. Then across to the big toes, up the front of the body staying inside the kneecaps and up to the front of the ribcage under the breast. Do the arms again.

Zip up front and back. Pubic bone up to the bottom lip, and tail bone up over the head, down the nose and stop at the upper lip. Do it three times.

Now repeat the whole process two more times.

Redefine your diet:

Keep drinking that water.

Today we are going to add juice. No, not store-bought sweet fruit juice. Cleansing, nutritious vegetable juice. Do you have a juicer? If not, see below. Want to get one? Let me recommend the one I use. It's the Omega 8006. I got it on sale on Amazon, and no, I don't get any commission or anything else for recommending it. I just love it.

If you have a good quality blender like a Vitamix, a NutriBullet juicer, a Nija juicer, or a Blendtec you can make juice, but keep in mind that the fiber is still all there, so it will be harder to digest and if you have issues with irritation in the colon, it is not the same as juicing. Some people use a blender and then strain out some of the fiber to make it easier to digest.

As a last resort use whole use juice powders from AIM or Juice Plus. Be careful, as a lot of the powders in health food stores are old, freeze-dried (which kills the enzymes), or contaminated. I have experimented with many and find AIM™ and Juice Plus™ to be the consistently good, alive juice powders.

The rule is five – you read that right, five – vegetables to one fruit. Some people juice by doing mostly fruit and then throwing in some carrots or spinach. When I say five, I mean five different kinds of vegetables and one fruit. So a handful of spinach, a large leaf of kale, half a long English cucumber, two radishes, three asparagus stalks, and a small beet + one apple = one large glass of juice. Drink daily.

Substitute any veggies you have on hand. Tomatoes, red or green peppers, zucchini, broccoli, cauliflower…if it grows on a plant you can juice it unless it is a grain.

Now you see why I suggest a really good juicer or using powdered juices. Blenders generally have a tough time with this unless it is one of the heavy duty ones.

It doesn't matter when you drink it, just get it done. Feel free to add parsley, cilantro, ginger and other herbs in very small quantities until you find your taste for them. There are lots of great books and websites on juicing.

Note: This is NOT a juice fast or cleanse, this is just replacing that afternoon snack or evening dessert with a juice. Your body will love you.

BIG HINT: Choose organic, locally grown veggies as much as possible. Grow your own. If you are concentrating the juice full of chemical sprays, pesticides, and chemical fertilizers, it is not going to do you very much good. Know your farmer and buy produce that is "spray-free" when possible if you can't get organic. Keep the *Dirty Dozen* and *Clean 15* list handy when you shop. It is updated yearly with which veggies are sprayed with the worst toxins and which ones are least sprayed and least likely to be toxic even when conventionally grown. The Environmental Working Group (EWG) puts out their annual "Shoppers Guide to Pesticides" report as well.

Restart your exercise:

Get out there for another 20-minute walk. Try to pick up the pace just a little bit. Walk out 10 minutes, going as far as you can, then turn around and walk back. Try to go fast enough to actually increase your breathing rate but not enough to get out of breath.

Release the toxins:

Today's toxin to be on the lookout for: **Phthalates.**

The problem is that most products don't say that on the label. They say "fragrance." Anything that says fragrance and does not also say from essential oils means it is the chemical phthalate family. Cleaners and laundry products are NOT required to list most chemicals on the label. They just put the ones they think you won't object to and conveniently leave the rest off the label under the claim of proprietary secrets.

If you are using any of the mainstream laundry detergents and softeners, you are getting a load full with every basket of laundry. Check your laundry – if you see the word fragrance, get rid of the products. Best plan is to dispose of it at your chemical recycling center; don't just dump it down the drain – after all, it is highly toxic. Next best, use it up and buy a better, cleaner product next time.

Want to know more, check out this article (I am not endorsing their product, but they do have a great short write up on the topic). Personally, I do use magnetic washing machine balls and occasionally a little natural, non-chemical soap when needed.

http://www.smartkleancanada.com/html/the_truth.html

http://www.womensvoices.org/

A great read on the topic is *Slow Death by Rubber Duck*; find it on Amazon.

—

DAY 3

There is no need to go to India or anywhere else to find peace. You will find that deep place of silence right in your room, your garden, or even your bathtub.

~ Elisabeth Kübler-Ross

Retrain your thoughts:

I have been telling my clients for years that you don't need to go anywhere to find yourself. You are inside. You need to peel off the grime, the cover-ups, the lies you tell yourself, the layers of guilt, and whatever else stops you from shining out.

Even five minutes a day of appreciation, mindfully enjoying yourself and doing something for you will help. Peace comes from the attitude of gratefulness and compassion within, not the activity or environment around you. Find just a few minutes a day to find your place of peace. Even if it is just sitting in your car quietly after you drop the kids off at school, before you go on to your next duty, relax, breathe, be grateful, let peace find its way from the inside out.

Reduce your stress:

Flip back and do the Meridian tracing again.

Some people find it best to do it in the morning as they get up and it gets them going for the day. Others like to do it at bedtime as it helps them wind down and slow the racing mind for sleep. Just do it. Of course, you can do it both times if you like.

Redefine your diet:

When I am at home, sometimes I juice at lunchtime. It's a nice break from my office on a paperwork day. If I am going to be out and about running errands, I take a shaker cup of filtered water and a container with dry juice powders and a dose of vegetable protein powder, mix and shake and have a nutritious lunch on the go. It's great for traveling as it goes through airports and I can always buy water if I have to. Remember, five veggies to one fruit. Any time in the day will do. For weight loss, replace a meal or snack with your juice; otherwise, just get it in you.

Restart your exercise:

Today you can walk again if you like, or if you are ready for a change or the weather isn't cooperative, try 20 minutes of yoga. All you need is a mat and the Internet. You can find lots of short yoga sessions and experiment with what you like. Just Google "20 min yoga workout for beginners" and you will find several great ones that will walk you through it step by step even if you have never done yoga before. It's a great stretching and strengthening exercise. Try it.

I know there are gurus who say it has to be done a certain way or at a certain time, and you have to do an hour with a warm-up and a shivasna to end. But in reality, just start somewhere. If you love it, and want to get into it, great. Otherwise get the value out of just doing. Pilates works too if you prefer that. Remember, just 20 minutes.

Release the toxins:

Today we are still looking for those nasty phthalates. This time look under your sink and in your bathroom for cleaning products that say the same things. The word FRAGRANCE is the code word for nasty, cancer-causing chemical. Of course, anything that says petroleum distillate is not worthy of your cupboard space either.

Replace them with vinegar and baking soda and elbow grease, since the exercise is good for you. Or explore your natural food store for non-toxic cleaners. There are some very good ones out there at about the same price. Check out "Method" brand, often sold in major grocery stores. Read the label…it looks quite different than the others but works really well. Natural orange oils and pine oils are the basis of many good natural cleaners. What you want to avoid are the petroleum-based ones and anything containing fragrance.

DAY 4

It is a not insult from another that causes you pain. It is the part of your mind that agrees with the insult. Agree only with the truth about you, and you are free.

~ Alan Cohen

Retrain your thoughts:

Sticks and stones may break my bones but names will never hurt me. That was the old saying back when I was growing up. And it is true – unless you believe what they say, it doesn't hurt. What others say about you or to you doesn't really matter, unless you agree with them and allow yourself to resonate with their words. Pouring hydrogen peroxide on healthy skin doesn't hurt, but pour it into an open wound and you will squirm. It is only when it is "true" in your own belief that insults hurt.

Using some of the exercises in Week 4 will help you undo some of the things you see as "true" that are not. Catching yourself in those beliefs and identifying them is a good place to start right now. Raising your belief in yourself, releasing the negatives and teaching yourself your real truth will prevent the insults from sticking. What untruths about yourself do you need to let go? Make a list. You will come back to it in Week 4.

UNTRUE BELIEFS ABOUT MYSELF:

1. _____

2. _____

3. _____

4. _____

5. _____

Reduce your stress:

Go back to Day 2 and do the Meridian tracing again.

Front, arms, back, arms, sides, arms, zip three times. Repeat the whole routine three times. Now wasn't that easier?

Redefine your diet:

Want to lose some weight? Try replacing one meal a day with a large glass of vegetable juice. You will be surprised how easy it is since the body is getting the nutrition it needs with less calories.

Restart your exercise:

Walk 20 minutes. Pick up the pace. Try to go one block further in the same time. Start out at a normal pace. At two minutes, pick up the pace until you have deep breathing. Keep it up until you are two minutes from home, then relax and cool down at a slower pace for the last little bit. Don't forget to drink a big glass of water when you get in.

Release the toxins:

Today's toxin is sodium laurel (or laureth) sulfate. In fact, it is a whole family of chemicals with many varieties in the name. If the initials are SLS, you don't want it. It is what makes things foam up and make a nice lather. Yes, it feels nice and makes you think the product is doing more good because it lathers up, but that is its only purpose. It doesn't actually make the product work better – it just meets our cultural belief that foam is better. On the other side, according to the Environmental Working Group's *Skin Deep: Cosmetic Safety Reviews*, research studies on SLS have shown links to:

- Irritation of the skin and eyes

- Organ toxicity

- Developmental/reproductive toxicity

- Neurotoxicity (brain toxin), endocrine (hormone) disruption, ecotoxicology, and biochemical or cellular changes

- Possible mutations and cancer

If you visit the SLS page on the Environmental Working Group's (EWG) website, you will see a very long list of health concerns and associated research studies.

Check out Dr. Mercola's lengthy article on it. Just Google "Mercola SLS" and it will show up.

Better safe than sorry, so begin replacing every product in your house that contains SLS. Start with the bathroom and laundry.

We will get to personal products next week. Think about what your office has. What about the toxic liquid hand soaps in the washrooms?

—

DAY 5

The part can never be well unless the whole is well.

~ Plato

Retrain your thoughts:

I love the fact that we are getting back to the wisdom of the ancients. We have lost our way in modern society, modern medicine particularly. We need to get back to the idea that all of me matters. I can't fix a pain here without addressing the misuse there or the lack of nutrition in food. If we want to be healthy, we have to look at body, mind, spirit and environment. Sticking Band-Aids on or medicating symptoms without addressing the thoughts and the diet and the stress has proven to be detrimental. That is why we have five strands to kick-start your new lifestyle. A lifestyle isn't just one aspect. You can exercise all you want, but if your diet is garbage, you cannot be healthy. Your thoughts lead to your beliefs, which lead to your choices, which lead to your actions, which determine your health. No matter how fast or slow you go at it, keep on the journey and the strands will meld into a path for life.

Reduce your stress:

Do that Meridian tracing one more time. It's getting to be smooth and easy now. Keep it up.

Redefine your diet:

What did you juice today? I had cucumber, red chard, aspara-gus, tomatoes, a large handful of parsley, red pepper, two handfuls of mixed salad greens, three carrots, and a mango. Delicious…and that is what was in my fridge.

Restart your exercise:

Today you have a choice of 20 minutes of yoga or try out the Tibetan 5s. There are many versions of it around. A quick and easy free one is found on Wikipedia. I don't often like Wikipedia because it censures natural health information and has a lot of "critics" or "scam-busters" who think they know a lot more than they do and who remove information posted by many credible people, but that is a different story.

In this case, they have nice graphics and short explanations of how to do them. Just search "Tibetan 5 Rites" and it will come up. You can skip all the history and the dispute about who should get the credit and scroll down to the 5 Rites. Very simple, deceivingly so. It's a lot harder to actually do 21 of each than it looks. Just do as many as you feel comfortable with and build up as you are able. Check out the appendix for instruc-tions if you don't internet access.

If you can't do Rite 4, don't be surprised or discouraged. That is a tough one. Start out doing a Little Bridge instead. Lay flat with your arms at your side and bring the knees up with your feet close to your buttocks. Raise your hips while keeping your shoulder blades flat on the floor. Hold for a count of five and lower slowly.

If you want to do this instead of walking or yoga, feel free. The benefits most likely to be achieved are increased energy, stress reduction, and an enhanced sense of calm, clarity of thought, increased strength and flexibility, resulting in an overall improvement in health and well-being.

Just do something.

Release the toxins:

Many of us are quick to grab the Raid or other toxic chemicals when we see ants, wasps, spiders, and other critters. We also grab the Roundup or Killex when there is grass or weeds growing somewhere we don't want it.

Take a second thought. If it is so toxic to them and to our pets, what it is doing to us?

Take a look at your garden supplies and your bug sprays. Most of them also kill honey bees. With bees dying off in alarming numbers we need to be careful what we spray. No bees means no pollinated foods. Are you willing to live without tomatoes, blueberries, strawberries, apples, peaches, and an endless list of foods that depend on bees for pollination?

Getting rid of weeds around the house is easy. Vinegar with a little dish soap sprayed or poured on the weeds will kill them from the roots. Want to kill grass permanently? Vinegar with salt in it will prevent anything from growing there. Use a ground cloth with mulch to prevent growth.

There are a lot of non-toxic bug approaches too. Check out www.eartheasy.com for great ideas. One of my favourites is for aphids. If your tree or garden is plagued with aphids put out a few small glass jars with apple cider vinegar (the real raw stuff) with a little dish soap. The apple cider vinegar attracts them in, the soap coats them so they can't fly away and they drown in it. Within a week, most of the aphids will be gone. Do it early in the season and you won't have a problem.

DAY 6

Be who you are and say what you feel because those who mind don't matter, and those who matter won't mind.

~ Dr. Seuss

Retrain your thoughts:

At first it can be hard to speak your truth. It may mean that the life you have been living will be exposed as a false front. Speak your truth kindly, non-judgmentally, calmly, but firmly. Don't hang onto something you don't believe for the sake of a community of people who are more interested in your compliance than your wisdom. As you grow, change, find your feet and become your inner self, you will find some new friends and others will drop away as you accumulate a new circle of people who are more in tune with where you are. It is OK to change circles and find those that affirm who you want to be. The old saying is you become the sum of the 10 people you hang around the most. Choose who those influences will be and let go of the people who mind that you are changing.

Reduce your stress:

Meridian tracing should be just about second nature by now. Notice how good it makes you feel. Pay attention to how it changes you and helps you center and focus.

Redefine your diet:

Today is farmers' market day for many (at least if you started on a Monday). What new veggies will you try this week? Add something different to your juice. Talk to your farmers' market people and find out where they get their produce. Who grows it and how clean is it? When you live in the north like I do, during winter a lot of "farmers' market" produce is bought from big warehouses and is the same thing you get in a grocery store. Don't assume they get better quality if the environment doesn't allow them to grow in the winter. Ask questions and get answers. Many of the large farms, including Hutterites and other Colony groups, sell at the markets but grow in conventional chemical large-scale operations. Don't assume that it is clean food. Ask if they use commercial feed for their animals and chickens. Ask what kind of weed control they use. "Organic" is becoming a big marketing feature and not everyone who sells at a farmers' market sticks to the clean growing that organic should have.

Restart your exercise:

You are in for a surprise today. This is your tough exercise day. Drum roll please…Introducing intensive interval training. Today is 20 minutes again. You will do this only once a week. If you want all the research on it, check out Dr. Mercola's exercise website or read *The 4-Hour Body* by Tim Ferris. For the fast version, once a week you need high-intensity intervals with rest periods in between to get your metabolism going. If you have a bike, stationary or free-wheeling, if you have some weights, great, but if not, don't jump ship and excuse yourself. All you really need is a street with light posts regularly spaced. If you can't do that in the winter, then some floor space with a mat will do.

The goal is to get your heart rate up to about 120 for 90 seconds, take a slower pace and let it lower for 2–3 minutes, and then repeat the cycle 8 times.

If you have a bike, crank up the resistance and pump hard for 90 seconds, slow down for 2 minutes and then crank it up again.

If you have weights, use the heaviest weight you can with the lowest number of very slow, controlled repetitions to get exhausted muscles within 90 seconds then, use a very light weight, but keep the pace very slow and controlled. Repeat 8 times.

If you can run outside, run as hard and fast as you can from one light post to the next, then jog slowly to the next one, then run like crazy again to the next one. Keep going for 12 minutes and then do a slow jog or walk home.

If all else fails, do a plank and hold it for 90 seconds and then run in place slowly for 2 minutes. Do another 90 second plank and keep repeating. You can use fast sit-ups, crunches, jumping jacks or anything else that will get your heart rate up and your muscles straining.

Anything will work as long as you get your heart rate way up, rest, get it up again and repeat the cycle.

Release the toxins:

Today's toxin is chlorine, also known as bleach. Chlorine has so many avenues of exposure. Scouring powders, toilet bowl cleaners, mildew removers, laundry whiteners, and household tap water give you exposure through fumes and possibly through skin when you clean with it. Because it's also in city water to get rid of bacteria, you often get high levels when you take a shower or bath. The health risks from chlorine can be acute, and they can be chronic. It's an acute respiratory irritant, but the chronic effects are less well known: it's a serious thyroid disrupter. Of course, it also ends up down the drain and damages aquatic life and fish habitat.

Ditch the bleach and use an oxygen-based cleaner. For scrubbing, stick to Bon Ami or baking soda. Toilet bowls can be cleaned with vinegar, and vinegar or borax powder both work well for whitening clothes. So does the chlorine-free oxygen bleach powder made by Biokleen. To reduce your exposure to chlorine through tap water, install filters on your kitchen sink and in the shower.

<hr>

DAY 7

Don't waste words on people who deserve your silence. Sometimes the most powerful thing you can say is nothing at all.

~ Mandy Hale

Retrain your thoughts:

Having lived many years in South America, for me the concept that defending yourself implies guilt is well ingrained. Subconsciously, we feel that we have to explain why we are doing something and need to have an excuse that is "good enough" for others. That implies that they have the right to judge us and our decisions. We think we have to have a good reason to say no or we will disappoint or upset others. Sorry, but I am not responsible for your response to me. If I say no, or, "Sorry, I can't attend," then my word is all that is needed. I don't have to explain myself to anyone.

Many things simply don't deserve a response and my silence allows me to stand in integrity and not be drawn into drama. Don't feel pressured to explain and make anyone feel better. Stand in your integrity and simply say no and be silent.

Reduce your stress:

Relax into your Meridian tracing one more time. Feel the flow and get used to the calm feeling it brings.

Redefine your diet:

Keep up your water intake. Remember that coffee, tea, or juice, particularly if it contains milk or sugar, does not count as water.

Enjoy a fresh veggie juice as a pick-me-up in the evening. It will help you avoid the evening snacking.

Restart your exercise:

It is your choice today: Walk, yoga or Tibetan 5s. 20 minutes.

Release the toxins:

What do you wash your floor with? I recently bought one of those floor steamers. It has a washable pad and uses just water. I love it. No chemicals, no refills or disposable pads for the landfill, just good old-fashioned water that steams up the dirt and cleans the surfaces. What can you do to reduce the chemicals in your home?

Week 2:
I create my future

We choose to be offended, when we could have made a different choice.

Other people aren't the reason for your irritation. The point of irritation is in you, and they have set it off. If it weren't them, it would be somebody else. They didn't bring irritation to you and dump it on you. Irritation is already in you; they just bring it out!

Well, you need to thank God that someone is bringing it out because when you recognize it, you can get rid of it. But you can't blame others, "He makes me so angry!" No, he doesn't. He calls up in you what shouldn't be there! Recognize it for what it is.

~ Graham Cooke, Seasoned in the Prophetic

This week will bring up the first of our modern society's approved addictions. As you deal with the physical level of food, you will also deal with the emotional level of letting go of old beliefs that no longer serve you.

In "Redefine your diet," we are looking at wheat and gluten.

I don't intend to write an expose or a scientific treatise on wheat. There are plenty of those available. Check out *Wheat Belly* or *Grain Brain* or hundreds of sites on the Internet about the dangers of modern wheat. Unless you are a celiac, I am not suggesting you go totally grain-free, though after you feel the difference you might choose to do so.

As a general disclaimer, I am not a qualified nutritionist; however, I am a qualified natural health practitioner and have seen thousands of cases of wheat intolerance, wheat protein allergy, and general inflammation caused by diet. Some general guidelines will help everyone.

No matter who you are, wheat, and grains in general, are acidic and inflammatory! It causes inflammation no matter who you are. So it's best to cut down on the quantity and ensure that the grain you are eating is grown and prepared appropriately. Using sprouted grains significantly reduces their natural acids, so that is a good starting point. Using them as a whole food rather than as refined food is another common-sense approach.

Throughout the week we will look at how what we believe shapes who we become. We create ourselves through our beliefs, our choices and our actions. From the food we eat and the things we put on ourselves, to our emotional choices, we create who we are.

I know it can get overwhelming and there is a lot of information and choices. You just do the best you can. Make a small step. Make one change. Eliminate and replace one product. Then, next month, cycle back and do one more. Keep building, keep expanding and it won't be long until you have achieved what you want to achieve. Focus on this as a lifestyle, a pathway for your life. This is not a 30-day diet or a boot camp. This is permanently redirecting your life. You create your future one choice at a time.

DAY 8

The secret of change is to focus all of your energy not on fighting the old, but on building the new.

~ Socrates

Retrain your thoughts:

Long before *The Secret*, Socrates had it figured out. Stop focusing on what you don't want and start doing what you do want. Just because something has been that way your whole life doesn't mean it has to stay that way or that there is a good reason for it being that way.

Let me tell you a story. My son has been taking a program at his college that includes online learning modules that apparently have to be completed within a certain time period or the program shuts down and you lose what you have done and fail the assignment. It forces students to work very quickly and often results in a great deal of frustration when he doesn't get quite done and it times out. He discussed it with the teacher and wanted some grace considering his learning needs. The teacher said the program has the time-outs and there is nothing he can do…too bad if you fail. However, my son also talked to the IT guy to ask if there wasn't some way around that. (Aside: Teaching kids to advocate for themselves is really important.) He was told by IT that actually there isn't a set time limit, it just times out because the government's Internet services are crappy and get overloaded. IT suggested he print out the module, do all the work on paper, then just go in and enter the answers quickly.

The pattern had been going on for so long and with so many students complaining that the teachers just assumed it was meant to be that way. How many things are you fighting that don't need to be fought? Find a way around the wall and build a new path. Don't take, "It's always been that way," as the answer. Find what works for you. Seek unusual allies. Build a new way.

Reduce your stress:

Keep doing your Meridian tracing. It only takes about 90 seconds now that you have the routine down.

This week we will add some meditation to move you to the next level. By meditation I am not referring to seeking to be nothing. The kind of meditation we are striving for is to quiet your mind long enough to listen to your heart and notice what your body wants to tell you.

This is my personalized technique. Hope you enjoy it as much as I do.

Linda's Body Relaxation Technique

Everyone holds stress differently in the body. Some hold it in the neck and get tension headaches; others hold it in the shoulders and get a sore back. Where do you hold your tension? It may be that you hold it in more than one place. Releasing built-up stress from the muscles and cells throughout the body can help you feel significantly better. It also strengthens your immune system and makes you less susceptible to "bugs" that are going around. It will make you happier too.

So pull up a comfy chair, put your feet up if you like, and shut off your phone for 15 minutes. Put a timer on for 15 minutes so that you don't have to look at your watch. Just do the exercise until the timer rings.

1. Find a comfortable position and allow your body to settle into your chair or couch. Close your eyes. Let your body melt into the chair and be fully in contact with it. Feel yourself supported and held up by the chair rather than just sitting on the chair.

2. Starting at your feet, slowly scan all of your body right up to the top of your head. Notice where you feel tight or tense.

3. Focus on your breath. Pay particular attention to how you are breathing: how quickly and deeply you breathe. Begin to inhale and exhale through the nose. Don't force the breathing or hold it out longer. Keep your mouth softly closed. Keep your jaw relaxed.

4. Become more aware of your breathing by paying attention to where your body moves with each breath and where it may be stuck and not moving. Feel the oxygen moving through your whole body. Let your diaphragm do the breathing for you. Feel your lungs filling up and pushing your abdominal area down. Feel your body absorb oxygen on the inhalation. On the exhale feel the blood releasing stress and toxins into the lungs and push them out.

5. Let the breathing and oxygen flow. Relax your whole body. Feel where it may be stuck or tight and send oxygen to that point until it opens up and moves with the breathing. Scan your body again to find any tight/tense spots and breathe into them until they relax.

6. At the end of 15 minutes, breathe deeply and slowly three times. Each time, as you inhale, feel your breath going all the way down to your toes and fingertips and as you exhale, flush out any tightness that may be left. Pause, and when you are ready, open your eyes.

Redefine your diet:

Your goal this week is to significantly cut down the white, refined flour from your diet and, of your sprouted or whole grains, reduce the overall quantity by 50 percent. If you usually have toast for breakfast and a muffin or bagel later in the day, cut out one of them and replace it with vegetables and fruit or nuts and seeds. Or if you are accustomed to eating two pieces of toast, make it just one. If you usually have a sandwich for lunch, make it a salad by leaving off the bread, and having some nuts with it or just a few rye crackers and hummus or avocado with it.

Go through your cupboards and fridge/freezer and take out everything that is made with processed white flour. On the label it may say wheat, wheat flour, flour, wheat starch or other terms used to deceive. If it is really whole wheat, it will say that. If it is sprouted it will say that. Otherwise it is just processed white flour. Check crackers, noodles, sauces, soups, and anything that isn't a real, natural food.

Make a list here of what you want to replace with a non-grain and which ones you will eat less of.

	Replace	Eat less
1.		
2.		
3.		
4.		
5.		
6.		

Restart your exercise:

This week is very easy. You have three choices that you can cycle through or stick to one for six days, and one day of intensive interval training. You choose which day you will do which one. Make a schedule now for this week. Your options are walking, yoga, or Tibetan 5s, 20 minutes each day. Ready, set, go….

Release the toxins:

This week we are looking at personal care products such as soaps, creams, lotions, face products, shampoos, anything you put on your skin or hair. I am kind of an earth mama and don't use very much makeup. I am not a makeup artist. I choose not to mostly because the majority of it makes my skin crawl. However, I know many people use a lot. The average adult in Canada uses eight products a day between body soap, deodorant, perfumes and colognes, shampoo and conditioner, liquid hand soap, hand sanitizer, and hair gels. Women use as many as 24 when you add makeup.

So here is the challenge. Go through the things you use every day and get rid of every one that uses the word "fragrance" on it. Set it aside and determine that you will find a replacement for it that doesn't have fragrance or any of the other chemical nasties you will learn about this week.

Remember the list of chemicals from last week in all the cleaners? Well, they are in your body products too. It takes 26 seconds to get from applying it to your face to arriving in your liver to be metabolized. My personal rule of thumb is, if I wouldn't eat it, I won't put it on my face. It gets into your blood stream just as effectively by being absorbed from the skin as it does via the mouth.

Remember, they don't have to put most of the garbage on the label so when you find the offending words, that is just the code for "lots of crap in here."

DAY 9

Some of us need to discover that we will not begin to live more fully until we have the courage to do and see and taste and experience much less than usual...And for a man who has let himself be drawn completely out of himself by his activity, nothing is more difficult than to sit still and rest, doing nothing at all. The very act of resting is the hardest and most courageous act he can perform.

~ Thomas Merton

Retrain your thoughts:

I need this reminder regularly. It is so easy to get drawn into being busy for the sake of being busy or worse, for the sake of someone else. Most people find ways to stay busy because sitting with our own thoughts and having to explore or even just be OK with what we find inside ourselves is not comfortable. It is impossible to be at peace with the world when you are not at peace within yourself. If your mind and your heart are at odds, your emotions are a roller coaster, and your thoughts run tapes of self-condemnation, then you will radiate those waves out and attract others who are the same and the inside becomes the outside. To change the outside, change the inside. To change the inside, you need to turn off the outer stimulus and learn to be at rest with yourself. If you can't enjoy time alone with yourself, why do you think others will enjoy time with you? Learn to be at peace, at rest with all people, especially yourself.

Reduce your stress:

Try that body relaxing meditation from yesterday. Learn to feel yourself from the inside. Allow yourself to be aware of how you are feeling, where you are holding your stress and feel how relaxing it is to acknowledge it, feed it oxygen and let it melt away.

Redefine your diet:

A major source of wheat is pasta and noodles. Try using spelt noodles instead. You can also buy green bean noodles at the Chinese grocers. Even better yet, use spaghetti squash. You can grow your own if you have a patch of sunny ground. It is the big, canister-shaped yellow squash. When cooked, it comes out in strings, just like spaghetti.

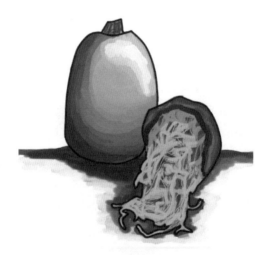

Spaghetti squash

If you want to get fancy, you can buy a raw food spiral grater (a little machine) that turns raw zucchini into "noodles." They are actually really good.

Restart your exercise:

Try walking today. Keep the pace up, but today, pay attention to nature around you. Don't just look at the houses and cement where your feet are walking – look to see how many different kinds of trees you pass. Look to see how many kinds of flowers you can spot. Listen for birds. Notice the butterflies. Connect with the real world as you are walking through it.

Many people put on headphones and music, or talk and walk without paying any attention to their surroundings, just getting the exercise done and multi-tasking. Let nature be your music. Give your mind a break and just notice nature around you. Twenty minutes isn't very long and you will survive without your headphones. If the traffic is too loud, find somewhere else to walk. Back alleys, pathways, and parks are good starters for you to notice what is growing, green, moving, and making the music of nature. However, do be careful and choose safe alleys to walk in. Know where you are going.

Release the toxins:

Today's toxin is **propylene glycol or butylene glycol**. It is a by-product of diesel fuel production.

It is linked to possible brain, liver, and kidney abnormalities, respiratory and throat irritation, central nervous system depression, pulmonary edema, brain damage, hypoglycemia, skin rashes and dermatitis. It is a neurotoxin that weakens protein and cellular structure. It is used as a cheap substitute for vegetable glycerin. It is often disguised as "humectant" (retains moisture).

Check deodorants, body lotions, body washes, hair conditioner, hair gel, creams, hand-wipes, and lipsticks.

It's banned in Europe, and banned in my house. Get it out of yours.

DAY 10

Don't underestimate the power of your own thoughts.

~ Louise Hay

Retrain your thoughts:

I love Louise Hay. I have lots of her books. Her down-to-earth wisdom and common sense is a breath of fresh air. This sums up everything she teaches. Don't underestimate the power of your own thoughts!

The tapes that play in your head…the subconscious beliefs you tell yourself…the doubts and fears that run riot in your brain, those are the thoughts that need to be brought into conscious captivity, forgiven and released. Need some help lassoing them in? Week 4 will give you some techniques to do that. Right now begin to collect a list of them. Write your own dirty dozen list of thoughts you don't want anymore. Catch yourself in the act and identify the lie. Many times just shining light onto darkness makes it disappear! The stubborn subconscious ones will need a little more, but shining light on them takes some of the power out of them and helps you see what you need to deal with.

And, it isn't the button pusher on the outside, it's the alarm on the inside that needs to be shut off and removed.

Reduce your stress:

Today try a variation of the meditation. We will again do 10–15 minutes but this time just observing your breath. The point is to quiet the mind and simply observe how the body interacts with the breath.

Sit still in your chosen position. Be mindful of your breath. Every time that your thoughts race off somewhere (and they will, along with song jingles, to-do lists and all manner of unwanted chatter), come back to your breath. Don't berate yourself if you begin wandering, just circle back to your breath.

- Breathe deeply in and out.

- Notice the different physical sensations you're experiencing as you breathe deeply in and out.

- Notice how your body expands as you inhale and contracts as you exhale.

- Experience the breath coming in through your nose, and out through your slightly parted lips.

- Experience how it feels through the rest of your body.

- Notice the stillness around you before and after each breath.

- Come back to your breath whenever the thoughts try to take over.

While it's important to try and keep focused, all beginners experience the inner chatter, the clamor of one's thoughts trying to regain supremacy and break the peace. That's OK. As thoughts enter your mind, just let them float out of your mind again and go back to focusing on your breath. This continual return to the present moment is the "practice" of meditation.

Attention may be increased if you ignore the inner chatter. The counting method is used successfully by some people. Start counting at the beginning of a breath meditation, counting for a few minutes. You will be focused on counting rather than other thoughts. Count each out-breath from one to ten, then return to one. Each time your mind wanders, return to counting again. Never overdo counting, though – it is possible to replace focus on the breath with focus on counting, and if that happens, stop counting and just notice your breath.

Redefine your diet:

There is a craze these days to go gluten-free and the marketplace is rushing to fill the gap with gluten-free products that look and taste like wheat or gluten, but aren't. Personally, I am not a fan of that. When you eliminate or reduce wheat and gluten, the point is to replace it with real foods like veggies, fruits and other live whole foods. Most gluten-free products are highly processed starches that are simply junk food without the wheat. Don't fall for it. There are some good gluten-free flour mixes for an occasional treat, but the point of reducing grains is to increase other food groups rather than replace them with more equally bad refined, processed, additive-heavy starch products. Reduce the grain but replace it with something colorful.

Restart your exercise:

Are you the one who likes to get a routine and do the same thing every day? Great, pick walking, yoga, or Tibetan 5s and stick to it six days a week. Do one day of high-intensity interval training and you are set for life.

Need a little more variety? Rotate the three however it feels good for you. Add Pilates if you like, just keep doing them. And, don't forget to work the high-intensity interval training into your weekly schedule.

Release the toxins:

Look for these in your products and get rid of them too.

PARABEN PRESERVATIVES OR ALKYL-P-HYDROXYBENZOATES (METHYL, PROPYL, BUTYL, AND ETHYL PARABENS)

- Hormone disrupter, estrogenic (mimics natural estrogens that lead to cancer); linked to breast cancer; skin rashes.

- Used as a germicide and preservative.

- Look for it in conditioners, hair styling gels, nail creams, foundations, concealers, mascara, facial masks, skin creams, and deodorants, sunscreen, and hair-colouring.

- It is banned in Japan and Sweden. Under review in the UK.

DAY 11

Life isn't about finding yourself. Life is about creating yourself.

~ George Bernard Shaw

Retrain your thoughts:

You are already on the right track here. If you have made it this far through the month, you are serious about creating a healthy, happy, focused, functional you. Did you know that in under three years, you are a completely new you? Not a cell in your body remains. You have replaced every one of them. So why do you still have the same problems and weaknesses? Well, damaged cells replace themselves with exact duplicates, recreating the problem. By changing the environment, providing better nutrition, doing the exercise and reducing the stress, you allow your body to heal and replace itself with healed cells. Remember it is not a race, it is a long-term commitment to creating yourself physically, emotionally, mentally, and spiritually. It is the rest of your life. You determine how it is going to play out on the stage of your life.

Reduce your stress:

Try the breathing meditation again. Set your timer for 15 minutes. The purpose is to gain control over the racing thoughts and allow yourself to actually feel and observe yourself. That alone will reduce the stress response in your body, lower your cortisol levels, and allow you to become more peaceful.

Redefine your diet:

What did you choose today to reduce wheat in your diet? One of the biggest temptations is coffee time. You feel the need for something and at the counter, what is handy is all wheat. Plan ahead and take an apple with you. The crunch will satisfy your chew reflex and the natural sugar and fiber will satisfy any hunger. Need a hit of protein? Dip your apple slices in almond butter or just munch on 10 almonds or walnuts with your apple.

Can't carry an apple? Take two tablespoons of chia seeds with you. Throw them in a bottle of water, and shake vigorously every few minutes. Wait 15 minutes until they have swelled up. Drink it down for a hit of protein, omega 3, vitamins and minerals and a full feeling. It's way better for you than a muffin.

Restart your exercise:

Do you pass near a nice park on your way to or from work? Take comfortable shoes and plan to stop and walk in the park for 20 minutes. Be mindful. Pay attention to the movement of the wind in the leaves, the variation of colors as the leaves flutter. Notice the bees on the flowers. Be grateful for bees that pollinate food for us. Notice the ants scurrying down the pathway. Get your mind off of work and other commitments. Be grateful to be alive and walking. Be at peace with yourself for 20 minutes. The pressures of the world will still be there but your response to them will be different.

Release the toxins:

Bet you didn't know formaldehyde had so many names! No matter what name, it is just bad for you. Reading labels is a survival skill these days. My general rule of thumb is if you can't pronounce it, it has more than four syllables, or it needs numbers as part of its name, it shouldn't be in your skin products.

Formaldehyde family, or Diazolidinyl urea, 3-diol Imidazolidinyl urea, DMDM Hydantoin , Quaternium-15, Nitropropane-1, Formalin, Methanal, Methyl aldehyde, Methylene oxide, Morbicid acid, Oxymethylene

- Is a suspected carcinogen that causes allergic reactions and contact dermatitis; headaches; irritates mucous membranes and damage to eyes, and is linked to joint and chest pain; depression; headaches; fatigue; dizziness and immune dysfunction.

- It is used as a disinfectant, germicide, fungicide, defoamer and preservative; it's cheap and mixes easily with water.

- Look in your shampoo, conditioner, shower gel, liquid antiseptic hand wash, skin lotions, bubble bath, hair care products, antiperspirants, nail polishes, talcum powder, mascara, mouthwash, and make-up remover.

- Banned in Europe.

—

DAY 12

You have to decide what your highest priorities are and have the courage—pleasantly, smilingly, non-apologetically—to say 'no' to other things.

And the way to do that is by having a bigger 'yes' burning inside.

~ Stephen Covey

Retrain your thoughts:

So what is your bigger, burning "yes"?

I have had this quote on my list of favorites for 10 years. I have changed the answer to it more than a dozen times. My yes changes with my focus and my clarity. I used to think that the bigger yes was something outside me. Something to do in the world. Something to achieve.

Now I have come to see that it is something to "be." It is inside me. It is my connection to the universe, to God, to Spirit. As that grows and is stronger and cleaner and less needy, I automatically do the things outside of me that result in something to do in the world and something to achieve.

My burning yes is being all that I can be and saying no to anything that takes away from that.

Reduce your stress:

Notice how having a purpose, a sense of being, automatically reduces your stress? When what others want from me, think of me, or say about me, doesn't matter, I have a lot less stress.

Let's try a meditation again that helps you keep the focus on just being and letting go of the attachment to all those thoughts about the outside world. Meditation helps to clean up the inside world.

Meditation is an approach to training the mind, similar to the way that fitness is an approach to training the body. Today's meditation starts by choosing a thought to focus on. It may be compassion, a prayer, a verse of sacred scripture, or a word like peace or joy. Just choose something positive that you want to develop inside yourself.

Find a comfortable, quiet place. Begin by simply observing your breath and relaxing the body. Notice any tension and send the breath there to relax it.

When you feel relaxed, begin to think your word. How does it make you feel? Does it bring up tension somewhere? Send breath there to relax it. Does it bring up thoughts? Let them drift away. Does it bring up images? Dismiss the ones you don't like and focus on one that embodies what you want to be with that word.

Spend 10 minutes or more just exploring how your body, mind, and heart respond and releasing anything negative while focusing on what you want to become through it.

Redefine your diet:

When eating out, ask the service staff not to bring a bread basket to your table. It is a lot easier to not eat it if it isn't staring you in the face. You could ask them to replace it with carrot sticks to munch on. If you are invited out, notify your hostess in advance. Or when you are out and you eat something just because it is served, then eliminate more at home to compensate. Remember, it is the overall quantity rather than the individual serving that matters in the long run. However, you may notice that after you eat wheat when you are out, you don't feel so well. As you eliminate it, your body adjusts and when you pollute it again, your body is likely to tell you it is not happy with what it got. Just saying…pay attention to how your body reacts to what you put in it.

Restart your exercise:

Is today a good day to do your high-intensity training? Max 8 cycles of 90 seconds with rests in between.

Release the toxins:

Here we are back as SLS again. A little more depth on why you need to get it out of your house and your body products.

LAURYL SULFATE (SLS), SODIUM LAURETH SULFATE (SLES)

- Can result in: suspected carcinogen-linked kidney and liver damage; nervous system disruption; damage to eyes leading to cataracts; eczema and dermatitis, known to inflame skin layers.

- Why it's used: foaming agent and emulsifier.

- Found in: toothpaste, shampoo, bath salts, body and shower gels.

- Banned in: Europe and Central America

Products without it may not foam as much, but is the foam really all that important? Foam is to enhance your feeling about the product, not to enhance its cleaning ability.

DAY 13

Fear does not prevent death. It prevents life.

~ Naguib Mahfouz

Worry does not empty tomorrow of its troubles. It empties today of its strength.

~ Corrie ten Boom

Retrain your thoughts:

Fear and worry are the two greatest robbers of all time. I learned a few tricks to deal with these a number of years ago. One of the easiest ways to lower your worry quotient is to keep a worry list and set a worry day. Choose one day of the week when you will let yourself worry – let's say Wednesday. The rest of the week, every time you start to worry, write the worry down on your worry list and then tell yourself, "I will worry about you on Wednesday." Now you don't need to remember it; it will get its time and you can go on with a clear head. On Wednesday, review your list and if you feel you really need to worry about some of the items give yourself permission to spend five minutes worrying about them. Most of the time, by Wednesday, the list looks quite silly.

Reduce your stress:

Remember to do the Meridian tracing. It will help you be calmer and more focused in your meditation.

Today, choose another word or sacred scripture and meditate again the same as yesterday.

Redefine your diet:

For a treat, try my gluten-free muffins. I make them with the pulp from juicing by separating out the strings and tough parts from the green stuff and keeping the pulp from carrots, beets, cucumbers and other soft-skinned veggies. It is high in protein and contains only good fats. Hope you like it.

___

CARROT MUFFINS FROM THE KITCHEN OF LINDA EASTHOUSE

Combine

1 cup raw creamed honey
1 cup melted coconut oil
1/2 cup olive oil
1 1/2 cup applesauce
2 tbsp chia seeds
4 tbsp egg replacer and 8 tbsp water (or use 3 eggs)

Combine separately, then add and mix well

2 cups flour (Use gluten free mix* if desired)
2 tsp baking soda
2 tsp baking powder
2 tsp cinnamon
1/2 tsp ginger
1/2 tsp nutmeg

2 tsp allspice
1 tsp salt

Add and mix gently

3–4 cups grated carrots, zucchini, beets, or any combination of veggies or use juicer pulp (remove heavy strings from celery or sharp bits like broccoli stem skins)
1/2 cup raisins or dried, unsweetened cranberries
1/2 cup dried currents
1/2 cup sliced almonds (optional)

Spoon into medium sized muffin tins. Bake at 350 F for 20 minutes or until a toothpick comes out clean. Makes 2 doz.

*Gluten free mix= 2/3 c coconut flour, 2/3 c garbanzo bean flour, 2/3 c rice flour. Mix and use instead of flour.

Restart your exercise:

You've been walking for 13 days now, or doing yoga or Tibetan 5s. How does it feel? Starting to notice changes in your body? Are you able to breathe better? Takes a little more effort to get winded? Maybe your clothes are starting to fit better.

A suggestion: find a walking buddy.

Release the toxins:

If you haven't seen this yet, you need to watch it. Did you know that on cosmetics, words like "natural," "herbal," and even "organic" are not regulated? They can say whatever they want and are not responsible to ensure they are true.

The Story of Cosmetics, released on July 21, 2010, examines the pervasive use of toxic chemicals in our everyday personal care products, from lipstick to baby shampoo. Produced with Free Range Studios and hosted by Annie Leonard, the seven-minute film by The Story of Stuff Project reveals the implications for consumer and worker health and the environment, and outlines ways we can move the industry away from hazardous chemicals and towards safer alternatives. The film concludes with a call for viewers to support legislation aimed at ensuring the safety of cosmetics and personal care products.

http://storyofcosmetics.org

And, for all you fact checkers out there:

http://www.storyofstuff.org/2011/04/1...

DAY 14

If you will change, everything will change for you.

Don't wait for things to change. Change doesn't start out there. Change starts within. And when you change, miraculously, your relationships, your health, your business, your children,

EVERYTHING else changes around you. But all change starts within you.

~ Jim Rohn

Retrain your thoughts:

Are you familiar with the concept of resonance? It is like the ripples in a pool of water. If you drop a stone in one end and someone else drops a stone in the other, the ripples eventually meet and become something different. When you change the size or shape of the rock or the angle at which you drop it in, the ripple changes so that when it meets the ripple from the other end, the meeting creates a different wave. Your job, your child, your finances may not have changed, but if you do, your rock changes and what you send out to meet those other things creates a different response. When the response is different, it allows the other rock space to initiate changes too. When you send out a different vibe, you get a different response. If you can stop dropping in rocks of fear and anger or frustration, then the other side will have the wiggle room to try a different stone. Your change affects them and causes changes in response. Be the change. The responses may be slow and almost imperceptible at the beginning, but others will respond differently and you will start to receive back a wave more in tune with your own.

Don't be surprised if as you change, some of the people dropping rocks in your pool decide they don't want to play anymore and leave. If they are unwilling to change their ripple, let them go. Find new people who want to play on your new wavelength. It is very common that as you grow and change, your circle of friends and acquaintances will revolve to accommodate those more in tune with the new you.

Reduce your stress:

Choose one of the three meditation styles and do it after you do Meridian tracing.

Redefine your diet:

Try one day grain-free entirely. Be sure to replace the grains with veggies, fruit, seeds, nuts, avocados and other healthy alternatives.

Restart your exercise:

If you haven't done your high-intensity workout this week, today is the day. If you have, congratulations and enjoy a mindful walk listening to nature and observing the plants and animals around you.

Release the toxins:

Head out to your famers' market or local healthy food store, armed with your list of chemicals:

- Lauryl sulfate(SLS), Sodium laureth sulfate(SLES)

- Formaldehyde family

- Paraben preservatives

- Fragrance (Phthalates)

- Propylene glycol

See what products you can find to replace the bad ones in your bathroom and home. You can also check out the Internet on formulas to make your own products with things like coconut oil, aluminum-free baking soda, essential oils and other natural pure oils.

Week 3:
I am what I eat

Today, more than 95% of all chronic disease is caused by food choice, toxic food ingredients, nutritional deficiencies and lack of physical exercise.

~ Mike Adams, the Health Ranger

Natural healing is about taking control of your life and being responsible for everything that goes in and out of your body, mind and spirit.

~ Richard Schulze

You are over the hump and halfway to the end of your first cycle. You are well on the way to creating the pathway to the rest of your healthy, successful life. You may not have kept up with everything but just do the best you can and then come back to repeat the cycle again. You can repeat it as often as you like. It is a manual and a plan. Keep following the plan, keep applying the instructions in the manual and you will build a solid foundation and create the life you want to have.

This week we tackle the toughest addiction you face. Yes, that is sugar. It is more addictive than cocaine and comes with so many emotional strings attached that freeing yourself from its grip will prove a challenge. But, you are up to it. You already have an established habit of calming your brain and exercising your body. That will prove to be a big support. You have lowered the toxic level of your body by cleaning up the chemicals. That will help your body free reserves to fight the insidious grip of sugar.

You can do it. One step at a time, one bite at a time, one day at a time. It's all downhill after conquering this one. See you on the other side of sugar addiction.

———

DAY 15

The 3 C's of life: Choices, Chances, and Changes

You must make a choice to take a chance, or your life will never change.

~ Daily inspirational quotes

Retrain your thoughts:

What choice will you make today? You have the choice to put something into your mouth or not. Yes, your emotional pull will seem stronger than gravity but in the end, you have the choice to simply close your mouth. You have the choice to make the changes in your emotions and subconscious beliefs that will allow you to make a change in what goes in your mouth.

Step one is plan ahead. Plan what you will buy. If you don't have sugar in your house, it is pretty hard to eat it.

Plan what you will take with you for your lunch or snack so that the sugar dragon doesn't slay you at your weakest.

Really get it into your head that your choice to take a chance on doing something different will help you make the change you want to see.

Reduce your stress:

PRACTICE DEEP BREATHING:

The key to deep breathing is to breathe deeply from the abdomen, getting as much fresh air as possible in your lungs. When you take deep breaths from the abdomen, rather than shallow breaths from your upper chest, you inhale more oxygen. The more oxygen you get, the less tense, short of breath, and anxious you feel.

- Sit comfortably with your back straight. Put one hand on your chest and the other on your stomach.

- Breathe in through your nose. The hand on your stomach should rise. The hand on your chest should move very little.

- Exhale through your mouth, pushing out as much air as you can while contracting your abdominal muscles. The hand on your stomach should move in as you exhale, but your other hand should move very little.

- Continue to breathe in through your nose and out through your mouth. Try to inhale enough so that your lower abdomen rises and falls. Count slowly as you exhale.

If you find it difficult breathing from your abdomen while sitting up, try lying on the floor. Put a small book on your stomach, and try to breathe so that the book rises as you inhale and falls as you exhale.

Just notice your breathing and do it for 10 minutes. Once you get into the habit, anytime you feel stressed, you can do a minute or two of deep breathing to turn off the stress responses and get more oxygen into your system, which will calm you.

Redefine your diet:

Today take an inventory of the sugar in your kitchen. Make a list, or better yet, pull out and put on the counter every item that has refined sugar in it. I am not counting pure raw honey, organic maple syrup, stevia, or other natural unrefined sweeteners.

Read the labels looking for sugar, glucose, and high fructose corn syrup.

Look again and check out this list courtesy of http://lowcarbdi-ets.about.com/ I edited the list to remove the unrefined sugars. This is just refined sugars that are the target of our campaign this week.

"Here is a list of some of the possible code words for 'sugar' which may appear on a label. Hint: the words 'syrup,' 'sweet-ener,' and anything ending in 'ose' can usually be assumed to be 'sugar.' If the label says 'no added sugars,' it should not contain any of the following, although the food could contain naturally-occurring sugars (such as lactose in milk)."

- Agave nectar
- Barley malt syrup

- Beet sugar
- Brown rice syrup
- Brown sugar
- Cane crystals (or, even better, "cane juice crystals")
- Cane sugar
- Corn sweetener
- Corn syrup, or corn syrup solids
- Dehydrated cane juice
- Dextrin
- Dextrose
- Fructose
- Fruit juice concentrate
- Glucose
- High-fructose corn syrup
- Invert sugar
- Lactose
- Maltodextrin
- Malt syrup
- Maltose
- Palm sugar
- Raw sugar
- Rice syrup
- Saccharose
- Sorghum or sorghum syrup
- Sucrose
- Syrup
- Treacle
- Turbinado sugar
- Xylose

Restart your exercise:

How far can you go now, compared to when you started two weeks ago? Have you improved your distance in the same time? Great. Keep it up. If you have been primarily walking, try the Tibetan 5s to gain more flexibility, or better yet, do both.

Release the toxins:

Today we start the process of getting the genetically modified (GMO in North America, GE in Europe) garbage out of your diet.

Just removing all the refined sugar will eliminate a surprisingly large component of the GMO foods from your diet. I am not taking about hybrid plants, just the ones created through gene insertion in the lab. Many plants like wheat are technically not "gene inserted" but have been chemically modified in a similar way and have become indigestible to most people.

Again, I am not going to go into all the science and debate about genetically modified (GMO) foods. They're commonly referred to as GMOs in North America but called genetically engineered (GE) foods in the UK and Europe. You can do your own research but believe me, from a health point of view, you need to keep them out of your diet. It is better to err on the side of caution than to be sorry later.

▬

DAY 16

You can't medicate your way out of a disease you ate yourself into.

~ Linda Orr Easthouse

Retrain your thoughts:

Are you taking any medications? What symptoms are they suppressing? Most of the medication taken by adults today is to deal with chronic disease. Those chronic diseases are primarily lifestyle diseases. Often you literally ate yourself into it, so you can literally eat your way out of it. Spend some time thinking about how you got into the state you are in now. What are the real underlying causes? Make a list of them. How many of them are emotional stress? How many of them are results of your pH being too acidic? (That includes inflammation, sore joints, weight gain, wacky hormones, blood sugar imbalance, heart disease, etc.) What do you want to do about that?

Reduce your stress:

I learned this years ago and don't know where the original came from. Thank you to the unknown originator.

Morning breathing

Try this exercise when you first get up in the morning to relieve muscle stiffness and get your system going. Then use it throughout the day to relieve back tension.

1. From a standing position, bend forward from the waist with your knees slightly bent, letting your arms dangle close to the floor.

2. As you inhale slowly and deeply, return to a standing position by rolling up slowly, lifting your head last.

3. Hold your breath for just a few seconds in this standing position.

4. Exhale slowly as you return to the original position, bending forward from the waist.

5. Carry on for several minutes.

6. Notice how you feel at the end of the exercise.

Redefine your diet:

Yesterday you identified all the refined sugar in your house. Today you are going to choose the top three offenders in your kitchen. Which of the products that you eat have the highest levels of refined sugar?

We are going to go at this slowly and take two weeks to get you off sugar. **Choose your three top sugar contenders and remove them from your kitchen.** Now find what you are going to replace them with – that is, a real, whole food that doesn't contain any refined sugar. For example, you eat corn flakes or Cheerios for breakfast. What could you eat that isn't cereal? Could you try a smoothie and some peanut butter on celery sticks? Who says breakfast has to be bread, cereal or muffins? Historically, breakfast was a protein meal. Be creative, find alternatives.

Restart your exercise:

Keep it up…now is not the time to quit. You've carved it into your schedule for two weeks now, so keep going. Little things add up. Instead of looking for the closest parking spot, take one at the far edge of the lot and walk at a good pace. At your kid's soccer game? Walk back and forth along the sidelines while you cheer them on. Every little bit helps, but don't give up on your 20 minutes a day. Keep it strong until it is a daily habit you can't do without any more than you would give up showering.

Release the toxins:

Aside from sugar, what GMO's are in your diet? Canola oil is the top offender in Canadian food. **Corn oil** is the top offender in American food, and **soy** in all its forms is everywhere.

Read labels and reject any food that list canola, corn, or soy unless they are listed as organic.

Next to sugar, canola, corn, and soy are the biggest GMO crops in our food chain. Most of them are mixed with wheat and sugar that you don't want either, so get rid of them all together. The toughest one is canola oil as it is used for cooking in almost every restaurant. If you eat out, you are getting GMO canola. Make sure you aren't also getting it in foods you buy at the grocery store or cook for yourself. Note: vegetable oil is a blend of soy, corn, cotton, and canola – all of them are GMO.

In North America, GMOs do not require labeling yet. You have to be vigilant.

DAY 17

The single largest predictor of a healthy diet is who is cooking your food. A poor woman who cooks at home is healthier than a rich woman who doesn't.

~ Michael Pollan, author of Cooked

Retrain your thoughts:

We have been so trained to think that instant is better. If we heat it up in a microwave, we think we "cooked" it. If it comes premade, ready to eat, we believe that if it looks good and tastes good, it is just as nutritious as if we cooked it ourselves but it saves us time and effort.

The problem is that it is not as nutritious. We gain empty calories, chemicals and toxins in return for time and effort. We become accustomed to food-like substances with unrealistic flavours that are intentionally addictive. We have to retrain our taste buds and our brains to recognize real food. We have to decide that it is important that we know where our food comes from and who cooks it and how it is done.

The cost of food is so high because there are so many middle-men and politicians in the food chain that the consumer and the farmer can't even find each other. We need to change our thinking and start demanding real, local, live food and begin to cook again. Teach your children to cook with real ingredients.

Reduce your stress:

Deep muscle relaxation – originally from the NHS in the UK

This technique takes around 20 minutes. It stretches different muscles in turn and then relaxes them, to release tension from the body and relax your mind.

Find a warm, quiet place with no distractions. Get completely comfortable, either sitting or lying down. Close your eyes and begin by focusing on your breathing, breathing slowly and deeply as described below.

If you have pain in certain muscles, or if there are muscles that you find it difficult to focus on, spend more time on relaxing other parts.

You may want to play some soothing music to help relaxation. As with all relaxation techniques, deep muscle relaxation will require a bit of practice before you start feeling its benefits.

For each exercise, breathe in as you stretch, hold the stretch for a few seconds, then breathe out as you relax. Repeat it a couple of times. It's useful to keep to the same order as you work through the muscle groups:

- **Face**: push the eyebrows together, as though frowning, then release.

- **Neck**: gently tilt the head forwards, pushing chin down towards chest, then slowly lift again.

- **Shoulders**: pull them up towards the ears (shrug), then relax them down towards the feet.

- **Chest**: breathe slowly and deeply into the diaphragm (below your bottom rib) so that you're using the whole of the lungs. Then breathe slowly out, allowing the belly to deflate as all the air is exhaled.

- **Arms**: stretch the arms away from the body, reach, then relax.

- **Legs**: push the toes away from the body, then pull them towards body, then relax.

- **Wrists and hands**: stretch the wrist by pulling the hand up towards you, stretch out the fingers and thumbs, then relax.

Spend some time lying quietly after your relaxation with your eyes closed. When you feel ready, stretch and get up slowly.

Redefine your diet:

The next step in your sugar purge is to replace all liquids that you drink, hot or cold, that contain sugar. Cold drinks can be replaced with plain water. For hot drinks, if you must add sweetener, use a little (focus on the "little") honey or stevia. Your grocery bill will thank you when you stop buying pop, energy drinks, sweetened juices, and other drinks.

Do NOT under any circumstances use artificial sugar. That would include aspartame, now called AminoSweet, Splenda, NutriSweet or any other artificial sweetener. One of the major problems with them is that they turn off the receptor that indicates you have had enough food. People who use artificial sugar eat more and drink more sweetened food because they lose the "satisfied" signal.

Of course, the fact that they are neurotoxic and cause your brain cells to literally explode would be reason enough to not use them.

Get used to drinking water! Purified, clean water is what your body uses best. Green tea, herbal tea, and unsweetened coffee in reasonable amounts are fine.

Restart your exercise:

On your mindful walk, if you come across a pond or lake with wild ducks and other birds, please do not feed them bread crumbs or popcorn. They will die from the lack of nutrition in it. If you must feed them, give them some raw grains, chopped-up kale and lettuce or other foods that they would naturally forage – never anything cooked.

Release the toxins:

On the theme of canola and soy oil, check out salad dressing labels. I'll bet nearly every one of them is made from canola and soy. Even the ones that say made with olive oil will have a small amount of olive oil and the rest canola or soy oils.

Be especially wary of "natural" brands. In today's unregulated foods, "natural" isn't legally defined, so they can use it to mean anything, hoping you think it means what we would normally mean. It doesn't; it is a code word for "genetically modified that we want to you think is clean."

It is really easy to make your own salad dressings. Use grape seed oil, as it will not thicken in the fridge, or make it in small batches with olive oil and keep it on the counter. The basic recipe is 1/3 oil to 1/3 vinegar to 1/3 water. Add spices, herbs, salt, and mix. The varieties are endless. Check out the Internet for all kinds of awesome recipes and just be sure to use clean ingredients and avoid the GMO oils. When using olive oils, go for the cold-pressed because they contain fewer of the chemicals used during the heating process where regular olive oil is extracted.

—

DAY 18

He who takes medicine and neglects to diet wastes the skill of his doctors.

~ Chinese Proverb

The doctor of the future will give no medication, but will interest his patients in the care of the human frame, diet and in the cause and prevention of disease.

~ Thomas A. Edison

Retrain your thoughts:

Both my kids were sickly as children. They had extreme allergies. They had repeated infections. At the beginning, even though I knew it was hurting them, I used the antibiotics and puffers. I was desperate with very sick kids, and I let the medical system put vaccines into them, until I saw the pattern. New vaccine, nose-dive in health, round after round of antibiotics, tonsils out, ear drains in, and then they would slowly start to gain ground again until we repeated the cycle. I started using diet and herbs early in their lives. We controlled sugar, removed dairy, did everything, but it was never enough. We lived in a rural area with a lot of agriculture. Back then they sprayed a lot. Come corn season, we had to leave the valley because of the allergies. We thought it was the corn, but now I wonder if it was the spray! At any rate, getting clean, non-GMO food, and avoiding the sprays, and other toxins is critical to some kids. Of course the real solution came when we were introduced to Health Kinesiology™ and sorted out the heavy metal contamination, the vaccine damage, and the allergies. Today with a great diet, they are doing really well. This isn't saying that medical intervention is never right. It has its place, but the doctors never told me there were any alternatives to drugs and surgery, which clearly were not working very well.

Reduce your stress:

This is a set of relaxation exercises you can do at work at your desk. Sit back comfortably; loosen any tight clothing if you can.

Start by connecting with your breathing for a few minutes. Just slow, normal breaths. Each time you breathe in say words to yourself such as "peace" or "relax." As you breathe out, tell yourself "release." Then start the muscle exercises, working around the different muscle groups in your body.

- Hands – clench one hand tightly for a few seconds as you breathe in. You should feel your forearm muscles tense; then relax as you breathe out. Repeat with the other hand.

- Arms – bend the elbow up and tense all the muscles in the arm for a few seconds as you breathe in, then relax as you breathe out. Repeat the same with the other arm.

- Neck – press your head back as hard as is comfortable and roll it slowly from side to side, then relax. Now forward, and roll it up to your ears. Now side to side, reaching the ear towards the shoulder.

- Face – try to frown and lower your eyebrows as hard as you can for a few seconds, then relax. Then raise your eyebrows (as if you were startled) as hard as you can, then relax. Then clench your jaw for a few seconds, then relax.

- Chest – take a deep breath and hold it for a few seconds, then relax and go back to normal breathing.

- Back – tighten your shoulder blades back and towards the spine, hold for three seconds and release. Then arch forward with the shoulders, lean forward and stretch out the lower spine.

- Stomach – tense the stomach muscles as tightly as possible, then relax.

- Buttocks – squeeze the buttocks together as much as possible, then relax.

- Legs – with your feet flat on the floor and shoes off if you can, bend your feet and toes upwards towards the shins as hard as you can, then relax. Then lift your legs up and stretch the feet away from you for a few seconds, then relax.

Then repeat the whole routine 3–4 times. Each time you relax a group of muscles, note the difference of how they feel when relaxed compared to when they are tense. Some people find it eases their general level of "tension" if they get into a daily routine of doing these exercises.

Redefine your diet:

How are you doing at getting sugar consumption down? As you removed the gluten and the GMOs, you have automatically cut sugar. The toughest ones to break are at social events where they are serving birthday cake or cookies, or staff meeting with muffins. Of course it is sugar, gluten, GMOs and toxins all rolled into one. You may just need to decide that one cheat event in a week is OK and not worry about it. Just choose which one you will allow yourself to indulge at. Don't be surprised when your body rebels and lets you know it doesn't like the cheat. Once you have that garbage out of your system you may find that it causes bloating, upset tummy, headaches, and more when you do eat it. Remember, you used to feel like that all the time and thought it was normal. Now you can choose to cheat and pay the consequences, but at least you know why you feel that way and know it will pass.

Restart your exercise:

Try taking the stairs instead of the elevator. Carry your own groceries. You can think of them as barbells. Get out and play with your kids. Join a community league. Go dancing. Help with the pathway clean-up. Do whatever you like that makes you move. The more you move, the stronger you get. The more energy you have, the better your metabolism runs. It's a vicious circle working to your benefit.

Release the toxins:

Take a look at the eggs, chicken and beef you eat. Where does it come from? One of the big box stores? Rest assured that it has been fed genetically modified feed, injected with antibiotics and growth hormones, given more antibiotics in the feed to allow for more animals per square foot and to increase weight on the animal. Beef has been fed grain to "finish" it with a good layer of fat. The problem is when cows eat grain that they were not designed to eat, their meat becomes more acidic and their fat turns from omega 3 to omega 6. Omega 3 is healthy, omega 6 is inflammatory. So yes, beef from the factory farm will make you sick because all the toxins put into the animal end up in the meat and the fat that you eat. Don't blame the cow, blame the corporate farmer. Find a real farmer who knows that cows eat grass and don't need extra hormones or antibiotics.

DAY 19

If you can't pronounce it, don't eat it.

~ Common sense

What you eat in private you will wear in public.

~ Unknown

Retrain your thoughts:

I have learned to trust my gut instincts and if my body says no, I need to respect that. Learning to read labels and recognizing that the real food is the ingredients has helped me make better choices. If food is made from non-food ingredients, it is non-food. I don't eat it. How about you? What are you learning to just reject? Going shopping is either very fast because I only buy fresh whole foods, or very slow because I read every label on the shelf until I find one that has food rather than junk. However, even real, clean, organic food eaten in oversized quantities isn't good. What you eat in quality and quantity shows in the long run.

Reduce your stress:

Try one of the meditations from last week or the tension-taming breathing routines again today.

Redefine your diet:

Keep vigilant and maintain your sugar strike. Your taste buds will begin to adjust and within 30 days, eating what you used to eat will feel disgustingly sweet and you won't want it anymore.

Use dried fruit, small amounts of honey, and real, raw fruits to satisfy the cravings in the meantime.

Restart your exercise:

Hang in there. You are almost to the 21-day mark, after which your muscles will actually start to crave the exercise and the stretch. Your routine will become more automatic. The payoff will start to show more. Need more variety? Try a different yoga routine or work out with a friend. Have a walk date instead of a coffee date with your friend.

Release the toxins:

RECOGNIZE FRUIT AND VEGETABLE LABEL NUMBERS

- If it is a 4-digit number, the food is conventionally produced with pesticide and sprays.

- If it is a 5-digit number beginning with an 8, it is GM. *However, do not trust that GE foods will have a PLU identifying it as such, because PLU labeling is optional.*

- If it is a 5-digit number beginning with a 9, it is organic.

USDA organic labeling may not be very clean. Big corporate interests have diluted it a lot. However, it does still require that the food not be GMO.

Canadian Organics are much stricter because it is run by the organic growers association and it is in their best interests to keep it strong.

DAY 20

It's bizarre that the produce manager is more important to my children's health than the pediatrician.

~ Meryl Streep

Retrain your thoughts:

Modern chemical medicine is the "alternative" medicine. It has only been around about 150 years. Our ancestors knew what the natural practitioners are trying to remind people of: food is your medicine. Clean up your environment inside and out, strengthen the immune system, provide real nutrition, deal with your stress in constructive ways, and the body will heal itself. It knows what it needs – we just aren't very good at listening or providing what we know. Old-school doctors used to tell their clients how to eat, what herbs to use, prescribe fresh air and exercise, and intervene with chemicals and surgery only when other methods had failed. If you break a bone, head straight to emergency. If you have chronic colds and flus, or high blood pressure, look at your diet and your stress. Remember, you can't medicate your way out of a disease you ate yourself into. Real, clean, food; pure water; and sunshine (if you live in the north like I do or under mostly cloudy skies, like in Vancouver or Seattle, you need Vitamin D, too). The best medicine is preventative.

Reduce your stress:

Which one would you like to do today? Deep breathing, morning breathing, deep muscle relaxation, office chair relaxation? It is great if you do more than one since none of them take very long. You can combine it with a meditation from last week and do your Meridian tracing at bedtime. Manage your stress throughout the day with little breaks to do these kinds of exercises.

Redefine your diet:

You will find store-bought treats such as cakes, cookies, and muffins, even if they are gluten-free, are much sweeter than ones you make at home. Find a recipe and simply cut all the sweeteners in half! Any recipe can be done with half the sugar and will still cook up and taste great. Once you have gotten accustomed to actually tasting the rest of the ingredients instead of just sugar, you will have a hard time going back to sickly sweet. Now that you are cooking with half the sugar, try replacing half of that with honey, or better yet, stevia. (It's also been suggested that you can replace some sugars with applesauce – even homemade apple sauce.) It still tastes great but reduces the refined sugars even more. Got picky kids who are addicted to sugar? Go at it slowly, reducing and replacing a little at a time as they start to adjust their taste buds too. Remember, you pay for it, so you get to decide what to buy. You are teaching them how to eat and cook for the rest of their lives.

Restart your exercise:

Want some fun? Look up Easter Bunny Yoga at MindBodyGreen. com. It can be done any time of year.

What is your alternative to walking when it is snowing and too cold or blustery and raining, or it's just too hot in the summer and you don't want to go outside? Have a plan, an alternative so you still get your 20 minutes of heart-pumping movement in. Some towns have a mall walkers' club where you can go and walk inside the mall before it opens and you have some company to walk with. Some large condo buildings have walking clubs and a circuit inside the building so you know how far you have gone. Live in a condo but don't have a club? Start one. It's a great way to get a buddy. Of course, it is best to be outside in fresh air and observing nature as you walk, but if mall walking or condo walking is the only way for you to do it, it is better than not walking.

Release the toxins:

Spoiler alert: You know the great little papayas that come from Hawaii? The little ones that fit in your hand and actually look ripe and taste great? Well, those are genetically modified to withstand high doses of pesticide and herbicide. So have a lot of pesticide and herbicide with your fresh fruit. No thanks! Don't eat them.

Time and again, the *American Academy of Environmental Medicine* (AAEM) has warned that GMOs pose a serious threat to health, and it is no accident that there can be a correlation between it and adverse health effects. In fact, the AAEM has advised doctors to tell their patients to avoid GMOs as the introduction of GMOs into the current food supply has correlated with an alarming rise in chronic diseases and food allergies.

DAY 21

A merry hearth doeth good like a medicine, but a broken spirit dries the bone.

~ Proverb

Better to eat a dry crust of bread with peace of mind than have a banquet in a house full of trouble.

~ Proverb

Retrain your thoughts:

The greatest diet in the world won't make up for overstressed emotions and a chronic stress load. Your fight-or-flight response to stress makes you acidic. Eating a good diet helps to compensate, but dealing with the stress is a lot better. Your stress response was designed to deal with immediate threats to your life, like a bear on the trail or a house on fire. You needed to be able to run, but then it was over, and your body relaxed. The adrenalin was used up and the parasympathetic response kicked in as you relaxed. Now stresses go on and on and pile one on top of the other, and they don't stop so the adrenalin keeps pumping. There is no running to use it up – before you get a chance to relax, the next stress alarm goes off. The chronic stress in our homes and jobs is flooding us with acids and creating an acidic environment that food can't keep up with. Yes, learn to eat right to alkalize your body, but better yet, learn to relax, turn off the stress buttons (more about that next week), and turn down the adrenalin. Remember, your reaction is what pushes the stress button. The situation may provide a trigger, put you are the one that pulls it. Take your finger off the trigger.

Reduce your stress:

Try a guided meditation. There are lots of good ones available on YouTube.

Find a quiet place, relax, turn off your phone, and just listen and watch.

TRY THESE:

Stress Gone in 10 Minutes by the TimeTrappers
https://www.youtube.com/watch?v=bhqU531xSN0
(10 mins)

30 Minute Meditation: Asking for Nothing .... And Receiving Everything by TheReachApproach
https://www.youtube.com/watch?v=NMldMnEfxX8
(30 mins)

Redefine your diet:

The question of candy needs to be addressed. Sugar-free gum is artificial sugar and kills your brain, while regular gum is sugar made from GMO corn. I guess it is time to give up that habit, unless you can find the sorbitol gum, which is only half bad for you.

On the other hand, nearly all candy is made from sugar, and mostly GMO sugar or high-fructose corn syrup, which is from GMO corn.

Chocolate is not all bad, if you are getting good quality dark chocolate (70 percent or higher) and it uses stevia or organic cane juice. Even so, small quantities are advised.

I have my own little treat for you. Try these to treat your sweet tooth.

—

LINDA'S RAW CHOCOLATE DROPS

In the bowl of your food processor:

2 cups organic raw cocoa powder
1/2 teaspoon pink sea salt
1/2 finely ground coffee (optional)
1/2 cup melted coconut oil
2 tablespoon melted organic butter
1/2 cup unpasteurized honey
1 tsp organic vanilla
1 cup coconut cream (the thick cream at the top of
the can of coconut milk--do not mix or shake the
can, open and scoop it off the top, leaving the liquid
on the bottom)

Pulse all the ingredients together. Continue mixing until chocolate mass forms and dough pulls away from edges of bowl.

Remove from processor into a shallow bowl, cover and refrigerate about 30 minutes.

With a teaspoon, scoop out and form rough balls. Roll in the flaked coconut. Keep in the fridge.

For rolling finished drops:

1/2 cup unsweetened flaked coconut
1/4 cup coconut sugar (optional)

Restart your exercise:

After a few of those chocolate drops, you may need to double your exercise.

If you have been doing the Tibetan 5 Exercises regularly, you should be up to doing 21 repetitions of each one. Try and speed them up. Doing more isn't necessary, but push yourself a little to do them faster. Once you have them down to about 10–12 minutes you can add some yoga or walking to keep the full 20-minute commitment.

Haven't tried them yet? Now would be a good time to give it a go, just to work some different muscles.

Tibetan 5 Exercises: http://en.wikipedia.org/wiki/Five_Tibetan_Rites

No internet, check out Appendix B for the instructions.

Wikipedia has nice graphics and short explanations of how to do them. Just search "Tibetan 5 Rites" and it will come up. You can skip all the history and the dispute about who should get the credit and scroll down to the 5 Rites. Very simple, deceivingly so. It's a lot harder to actually do 21 of each than it looks. Just do as many as you feel comfortable with and build up as you are able.

If you can't do Rite 4, don't be surprised or discouraged. That is a tough one. Start out doing a Little Bridge instead. Lay flat with your arms at your side and bring the knees up with your feet close to your buttocks. Raise your hips while keeping your shoulder blades flat on the floor. Hold for a count of five and lower slowly.

Release the toxins:

Check out the Non-GMO Verified label. http://www.nongmo-project.org/

This is a non-profit organization that certifies a product does not contain GMOs nor has been produced using GMO ingredients.

Look for this seal on products to ensure you are getting clean food. Just because something says "no GMOs," unless it has this seal, it is just advertising. They can say what they want as GMOs are not regulated or labeled in North America. Join the fight in your country to force labeling rules that benefit the consumer and require honest, transparent labels.

Week 4:
I can stop the self-sabotage

You are in the home stretch now. It's amazing how far you have come in just three weeks. I know it has been a huge effort on your part. I also know you can't keep up a routine like this through effort alone. You need the mental and emotional shifts that turn this into an internal motivation because your burning desire is to have a balanced, do-able lifestyle where you feel in control and have your priorities and values running your life. Your family will run so much more smoothly when you are running smoothly.

This is about the point at which effort runs out of steam and you start self-sabotaging. You think, if I don't do my meditation and stress relief today, it will be OK. Or, if I skip the exercise for today it won't matter, I will get back to it tomorrow…but tomorrow never comes. Don't do it.

Self-sabotage can be such a subtle thing. It is rooted and grows from old patterns established when you were young or even inherited via your mother in the womb based on how she handled stress. But never fear, there are ways to deal with that.

This week you will learn some techniques to change your brain patterning and turn off the stress responses so that you can make better choices and still the voices of dissent from inside your head.

As well this week, we will tackle the issue of dairy. There is oh-so-much you think you know about dairy that is the result of clever marketing campaigns and not really true. Be ready for some surprises.

By now you might also be finding yourself a little overwhelmed with the pace of change, especially if you are trying to do all the strands at once. It is not too late to drop one or two of them and decide to repeat the process next month to fine-tune several of the strands and then pick up the others. This isn't a race. It is OK to decide you need to slow the pace. Just stay on the road and solidify the foundation. These are patterns for the rest of your life. If it only takes you two or three months to get them all into a smooth routine, you are doing great. For many people it will take five months to get the foundation laid and then a few more months to really get it automated. So just keep moving forward. Some things will feel like an uphill grind, others you will begin to coast with, and still others will finally click in and you'll feel the downhill wind. Enjoy the ride.

DAY 22

You will never change your life until you change something you do daily. The secret of your success is found in your daily routine.

~ John C Maxwell

Retrain your thoughts:

Some of us find routine stressful. Yes, I know that sounds crazy to a lot of people, but routine tends to bore me, and then I stop doing it. To master the steps of creating a life that is sustainable and healthy, there just has to be some routine. To keep myself on track I try to build variety into my routine: some days I walk in the afternoon, some days I do the Tibetan 5 Exercise when I get up, and other days I do yoga just for fun.

The same is true in other areas. Some of you will decide you like one of the relaxation or breathing exercises and just do it. Others, like me, will do these all a few times and then go looking on the Internet for something more. The point is to find your routine and do it daily. If you get the big rocks in the foundation, then the rest of the day will have more structure and you will accomplish the changes you want.

Reduce your stress:

Today I want to introduce you to one of my best practices. It is called the Emotional Stress Release. It is an easy Health Kinesiology™ treatment you can do for yourself anytime you are feeling stressed.

EMOTIONAL STRESS RELEASE™

Stress comes in many forms and from many causes, but in the underlying process, what happens is that the brain releases a storm of chemicals such as adrenalin, cortisol, and many others in response to what you are thinking and feeling. These bio-chemicals race around the brain and through the body, causing havoc. More than 100 chemicals in the body change when you are under stress. They can prevent you from thinking something through and coming to a logical conclusion by sabotaging your thinking and keeping you in a cycle of agitation.

This simple technique is like letting the stream valve off of a pressure cooker to let the steam out. It will take the emotional edge off of most stressful situations and allow you to move forward. It will not completely "fix" the problem that is stress-ing you but it will help stabilize you and allow you to get past the overwhelmed or stuck feelings so that you can deal with the issue.

Many different kinds of kinesiology have some variation of this correction. I find this one to be the most robust and the quick-est. While you are feeling stressed or emotionally overwhelmed, hold these points and think about whatever is stressing you. Normally you don't want to think about the "bad things"; however, while you are holding the points, you need to think about them so that the brain can shut down the stress response to them. You are accessing the circuits so that the points being held can "turn them off."

You will hold what are technically called the "neurovascular points, element 0, of the central and governing meridians." Don't worry about the name, just follow the picture below. You can do it laying down or sitting up. Many students and business people use it sitting at a desk, leaning on their elbows.

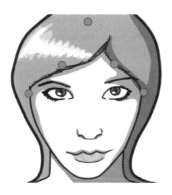

Hold these points for the ESR

1. Start with your thumbs just past the temple directly out from the corner of the eye.

2. Then put your little "pinkie" fingers on the forehead, one on each side directly above the center of the eye when looking forward, about halfway between the eyebrow and the natural hairline. If you put your elbows out in front your hand will twist towards the face enabling you to reach the points.

3. Put your second or third fingers together on top of the head on the soft spot.

4. Hold the points very gently, no pressure or rubbing required.

5. Think about whatever is stressing you until you feel better. It may be one minute, or five minutes, or half an hour, depending on how big and deep your stress issue is.

Redefine your diet:

Dairy is such a controversial topic. Let's start with some basics.

Milk (and therefore cheese, yogurt, sour cream, etc.) in the U.S.A. is very different than in Canada because of regulations around growth hormones and allowable limits. That said, neither are going to do you any good, with a few caveats.

Milk in North America is pasteurized at high temperatures. When milk is pasteurized, the calcium bonds to the protein and becomes virtually non-bioavailable. Yes, you read that right. Once it is pasteurized the calcium is there but your body can't take it out and use it. So all those ads about milk being a great source of calcium? Just marketing. Raw milk is a great source of calcium, enzymes and protein. Once you cook it at high temperatures, all you have left is the protein and the fat. Raw milk from cows that are fed real grass rather than corn-based silage, given no hormones or unnecessary antibiotics, and are treated well and kept in a field that has not been sprayed, is very good for you. A healthy cow in clean, uncrowded environments produces healthy milk.

So if you are drinking milk or milk products for calcium, don't bother. There are much better sources of calcium in green plants. After all, the largest mammals on the planet with the biggest, strongest bones get all their calcium from a diet of green leaves and grasses. That is where you should get yours.

If you need a milk-like product, choose almond milk, rice milk, hemp milk, flax milk, or coconut milk. Note: soy is not in the list for a reason. Drinking soy milk, organic or not, is not a good alternative. Soy must be fermented to be digestible and soy milk is not fermented. Choose one of the others and be sure to look for ones that do not contain sugar, carrageen, guar gum and other unnecessary additives that can cause digestive upsets. They are added to make it a more milk-like consistency.

Personally, I like homemade almond milk. It's super simple and delicious – all you need is a good blender.

EASY ALMOND MILK

½ cup almonds, soaked overnight. Keep the liquid from soaking.

Peel the almonds in the morning. The skins just pop off after soaking.

Put into blender with liquid.

Add 1 cup boiling hot water.

Blend several minutes until almonds are dissolved into the water.

Add 2 cups more cold water and blend another minute.

Strain through a fine mesh bag or coffee filter. (Health food stores often sell Nut Bags for this.)

Keep the pulp and add to baking instead of flour (freeze if you like) or throw into curry sauces.

Pour the milk into a glass bottle.

Add a pinch of sea salt and a teaspoon of real vanilla.

Keeps 2 days in the fridge, but it will be gone long before then.

Restart your exercise:

You have passed the 21 days required to form a habit! Don't give up now.

What will it be? Plan out your week: walking, Tibetan 5s, yoga, or a combination and one day of intensity training. Write it into your day timer.

Release the toxins:

In the first week you removed hormone-mimicking toxins from your cleaners. The second week you cleaned up your body products. Now, we are looking at where hormones lurk in your food supply.

Beef and chicken are both given hormones to increase the speed at which they mature and the amount of weight they gain. If you are buying beef and chicken from any of the big box grocery stores, it will have been given hormones. If you are eating at restaurants or buying at a meat shop, unless they say it is grass-fed and hormone free, it is not. Most restaurants and meat shops buy from the same slaughterhouse that supplies the big stores. The cows have an implant and the chickens get it in their feed. You get it from their meat. The only solution is to buy organic meat or get it from a local farmer who does not implant or use commercial feed that contains hormones or antibiotics. Beef must be grass-fed. Feeding it grain and corn is simply to fatten it up so they earn more from selling it. You don't need the omega 6 that is produced in cows that are grain-fed, but you do need the omega 3 that is produced by cows that eat grass. Local farmers' markets and farmers are good sources, but check what they feed. Just because meat is from a farm doesn't mean the farmer doesn't feed the animals commercial feed full of additives. Ask questions, visit the farm, and know where your food comes from.

DAY 23

An entire sea of water can't sink a ship unless it gets inside the ship. Similarly, the negativity of the world can't put you down unless you allow it to get inside you.

~ Goi Nasu

Retrain your thoughts:

We all have a frequency that we vibrate at. Just like a tuning fork will make a guitar string hum when they are exactly matched, the world's negativity will make you hum if you are matched to it. We resonate with the things outside of us that are already on the inside of us. If you are angry and people are angry around you, it just feeds your anger. If you are calm, the angry people around you can be brushed off and not taken personally. The trick is to work on getting the negativity out of you, so you don't resonate and reinforce it through your surroundings. Clean the inside and don't let the outside in.

Reduce your stress:

One of the ways to clean the inside is to shut off the tapes that run in your head and tell you things that are no longer true. You have beliefs about yourself that were often formed in childhood. They may have been a moment that got frozen in your psyche and now has generalized until you believe it about yourself. Maybe in a moment of frustration and anger you told yourself (or someone else told you), "I never finish what I start." That was about one specific event where you failed to finish something. But it got stuck, frozen in time. It grew until it applied to everything. Now, you have a subconscious self-sabotaging belief about yourself that prevents you from finishing things.

How do you get rid of it? Jimmy Scott, PhD and founder of Health Kinesiology™, created a wonderful little technique called **Belief System Elimination**, often referred to as BS Elimination. You can watch some demos of it on my website in the Resources/Self-help Video section.

BELIEF SYSTEM ELIMINATION:

To do it, you just need to identify the thought that is stressing you. Pay attention to the tape in your head that is sabotaging you and write it down. To correct it, you are going to repeat it out loud while you do little pinches at the hairline in the front (middle of the forehead) and sideways across the back of the skull where the spine joins the skull (about a half-inch wide pinch). Keep pinching lightly in both places while you repeat the sentence out loud for about 30 seconds to a minute or until you feel it change.

You can do one or two each day. Don't overdo it as you can cause yourself quite a reaction as your brain rewires those thought. Too many at once and you may feel very tired and even give yourself a headache until it finishes rewiring. Check out the appendix at the back for a full explanation if you don't have access to the video.

Redefine your diet:

Soy milk is not a good substitute. Soy is another dietary source of hormones. If you are going to eat soy, it should be fermented. Tempe, tofu, soy sauce and nato are all fermented soy and can be eaten in reasonable quantities provided they are organic.

Nearly 80 percent of all soybean crops grown in the U.S. are genetically modified (GMO), compared to in 1996, when only 7 percent were GMO soybeans. The great majority of soy today comes from Brazil, where GMO has taken over.

Unfermented soy is known to have a high hormone load. For centuries soy consumption has been associated with infertility. Couples struggling with infertility should not have any soy products. Pregnant women in the Chinese and Japanese cultures avoid soy because of the hormone disruption it can cause. On top of its natural fertility suppression, GMO soy is even worse because the modification affects fertility too.

The question of soy protein isolate for shakes is always a controversy too. It supposedly has had all the hormones removed and only protein is left. But on the other hand, how many of them are organic and not filled with the chemical contamination of sprayed, non-organic soy? They don't tell you. Then there is the issue of it being a highly refined, processed food-like product that the body may not really digest very well. Personally, I avoid it. Want protein? Get it from a plant-based powder that isn't so refined.

Restart your exercise:

Ready to push it up a little? Try doing two of the exercises a couple of days this week. Maybe do Tibetan 5s in the morning and do your walk, or do some yoga in the morning and a walk after dinner. Find a child, a pet, or a friend to do it with you. Have some fun with it.

Be careful that you don't undo the benefit of your exercise by having a high-calorie sugar sports drink afterwards. Just water works best. If you really need some rehydration salts, try AIM Peak Endurance or Zija Smart Mix for a quick refresher that is healthy, sugar-free and provides real nutrients. Be careful too of power bars and protein bars. They are usually high is sugars and carbs as well as a lot of additives – even the so called "healthy" ones. Eat a handful of nuts or an apple instead. You will feel just as satisfied and enjoy the benefits of your exercise more.

Release the toxins:

Reread the section above on soy. Soy as a whole food, properly fermented, is food. Soy protein isolates as found in soy burgers, fake meats, protein powders and baby formula is a high-processed, denatured protein that contains solvents, processing chemicals, and who knows what else. It is best left alone. If you are vegetarian, eat vegetables, not food-like products created in a factory.

—

DAY 24

In order to change we must be sick and tired of being sick and tired.

~ Anonymous

Retrain your thoughts:

It always amazes me how often I catch myself thinking, "I'll just put up with this." I let myself suffer and just get through it rather than make the choice to change something. Often a little change has huge results, but we let ourselves suffer through things until we get sick and tired of it and can't take any more...then we change. What a crazy way to do things! Yet I do it myself all the time. Somehow our culture has taught us that change is worse than carrying on with suffering. We think it is honourable to suffer and hold ourselves together rather than change. Why do we believe we have to hit rock-bottom before it is good to change? Step out, make the change early and cut the suffering. Why should I be sick and tired before I look for a way to be happy? That would be a good one to do for a BS Elimination.

Reduce your stress:

Try some more of the BS Eliminations. In the Appendix there is a list of common ones. Choose two that resonate with you and eliminate them. Watch Part 2 of the BS Elimination video if you haven't already done that.

Redefine your diet:

If you are feeling deprived with no refined sugar and no dairy, try this for a great pick-up.

—

FRUIT WHIP

4 cups frozen fruit chopped before freezing – mangoes, strawberries or pineapple work great.

> 1 cup coconut milk (shake can well to mix)

> 2 tablespoons of maple syrup or honey or use stevia leaves to taste

In a food processor blend the frozen fruit until chunky. Add the milk and sweetener and blend until smooth.

Serve immediately. You won't feel deprived anymore!

Restart your exercise:

What did you do today? No, walking all over Ikea doesn't really count as exercise, so choose a more stretching, relaxing exercise today to offset your sore feet. Build exercise into your chores. If you have to mow the lawn, do it with a push mower instead of a power one. Rake up leaves by hand instead of using a blower. Of course if you live in the north like I do, you can shovel snow for exercise most of the year. Just do something and try to enjoy it. You are much more likely to keep at it if you like what you are doing.

Release the toxins:

Since we are looking at hormones and toxins in foods and homes, have a look at the list in Appendix C. Today, we will start with **Sodium benzoate and potassium benzoate**. Check your kitchen. The obvious sources are plastic bottles with pop and fruit juices; in the fridge you will find it in many Asian sauces and hot sauces; and in the bathroom read labels to see how many products contain this one. When you replace them, buy products that don't contain either of these.

Sodium benzoate and potassium benzoate

These preservatives are sometimes added to soda to prevent mold from growing, but benzene is a known carcinogen that is also linked with serious thyroid damage. Dangerous levels of benzene can build up when plastic bottles of pop are exposed to heat or when the preservatives are combined with ascorbic acid (vitamin C). It's often found in fruit juices, even those marketed as "healthy." In the body it breaks down into formaldehydes.

Sodium benzoate is found in fruit juice, salad dressings, carbonated drinks (carbonic acid), jams and fruit juices (citric acid), pickles, and condiments. It is also used as a preservative in medicines and cosmetics such as shampoo, body wash and cleanser, facial cleanser, hair color and bleaching, facial moisturizer/treatment, mouthwash, anti-aging, liquid hand soap, shampoo plus conditioner, and hand cream.

DAY 25

I can feel guilty about the past, apprehensive about the future, but only in the present can I act. The ability to be in the present moment is a major component of mental wellness.

~ Abraham Maslow

Retrain your thoughts:

A lot of the stress release work we have been doing is to help you be in the present moment. From years of working with clients who self-designate as "depressed" I have come to recognize a pattern: avoiding living in the present because it is not what they want, pretending it is OK when it isn't, and surviving by living in the past or escaping into illness creates a deep and often unrecognized anger that is turned inwards. As that anger builds, depression is the illness of choice to repress it and keep it from bursting into the present. For it to resolve, it must be felt in the present. It must be accepted and released. Learning to stay in the present with your emotions is one of the most important skills you can develop. Emotions, any emotions, are OK. It is what you do with them that damages or fulfills you.

Reduce your stress:

One of best ways to get back into the present is to do the Emotional Stress Release while thinking about whatever you are trying to escape from. When you find yourself falling into stress or depression, there is a good chance that you are escaping the present. Allow yourself to be present and feel what you feel. Don't hold on to what you feel, just acknowledge it and let it flow through.

Redefine your diet:

We are still on the topic of dairy this week. If you are lucky enough to live on a farm and have a cow from which you can get raw organic milk, go ahead and drink it. For the rest of us, the process of pasteurization ruins the milk. So what options are available? For making creamy sauces, using in coffee and putting on cereal, try any of the nut milks you can make at home with a blender. Raw cashews make the creamiest milk. Personally, I use coconut cream to make sauces, soups, and curries. You can buy it in boxes with all the liquid removed so that things don't become watery. You can buy it in cans with the "milk" variety, which adds liquid. Experiment with a little at a time. It can be overpowering if overdone. In many places you can get flash-pasteurized goat's milk, which is suitable for many people, and because it is pasteurized at a lower tempera-ture for a very short time, sufficient to kill brucellosis but not enough to bind the calcium or ruin the enzymes, you get most of the benefit of the milk without any danger. Check your local farmers' market. The ones in your large box grocers are tradi-tionally pasteurized for longer shelf life – not good.

Restart your exercise:

Keep walking. Remember to be mindful and notice and ground yourself as you walk. Pick up the pace. Check back to Week 1. How far did you go in the same time then? I'll bet you get further now! Keep it up. Push yourself just a little each time. Stretch out your step a little. Good, just a shade faster. Every step counts.

Release the toxins:

MONOSODIUM GLUTAMATE (MSG/E621)

MSG is an amino acid used as a flavor enhancer in soups, salad dressings, chips, frozen entrees, and many restaurant foods. MSG is known as an excitotoxin, a substance which overexcites cells to the point of damage or death. Studies show that regular consumption of MSG may result in adverse side effects which include depression, disorientation, eye damage, fatigue, head-aches, and obesity. MSG affects the neurological pathways of the brain and disengages the "I'm full" function, which explains the effects of weight gain.

Found in: Chinese food (Chinese restaurant syndrome) many snacks, chips, cookies, seasonings, most Campbell's soup products, frozen dinners, lunch meats.

INGREDIENTS THAT ALWAYS CONTAIN MSG

- Autolyzed yeast
- Calcium caseinate
- Gelatin
- Glutamate

- Glutamic acid
- Hydrolyzed protein
- Sodium caseinate
- Textured protein
- Monosodium glutamate
- Yeast extract
- Yeast Food
- Yeast nutrient
- Monopotassium glutamate

INGREDIENTS THAT OFTEN CONTAIN MSG

- Flavors and flavorings
- Seasonings
- Natural flavors/flavorings
- Natural pork flavoring
- Natural beef flavoring
- Natural chicken flavoring
- Soy sauce
- Soy protein isolates
- Soy protein
- Bouillon
- Stock
- Broth
- Malt extract
- Malt Flavor
- Barley malt
- Anything enzyme-modified
- Carrageenan
- Maltodextrin
- Pectin
- Enzymes
- Protease
- Corn starch
- Citric acid
- Powdered milk
- Anything protein-fortified
- Anything ultra-pasteurized

▬

DAY 26

Your mind and body are linked, which can't be seen, but only felt. Your body reflects your emotional and psychological states. A positive mental attitude and powerful immune system will be the result of a healthy spiritual, physical and emotional state. It is only when we ignore our bodies that illness is able to take control of our own bodies natural defenses.

~ *Sam Tolman*

Retrain your thoughts:

Over the years of working with clients, it has become clear to me that we cannot separate physical health from emotional, mental, or spiritual health. We are unified beings and all parts affect and are affected by all the other parts. We talk as if there were actually separate parts, but there aren't. You are a whole being and different aspects can be affected differently, but none can be affected in isolation. If you want your immune system to function, then your emotions and your diet and your sense of inner peace all have to be working. Without the whole, any one individual system will burn out trying to carry the load. That is why it is so important to do all five strands: they work synergistically together to bring health.

Reduce your stress:

Do the relaxation exercise from Day 8. Notice how your body feels. Notice where you are holding your stress? Let it go. Where do you feel your worry? Where do you hold your guilt? See how your body, spirit, and mind are all intertwined. Relax them all.

Redefine your diet:

Family going out for ice cream? Choose a fruit gelato; check to be sure it is dairy-free but it does have a hit of sugar, so choose a small size.

Making your own at home. There are plenty of recipes mostly based on a coconut milk, banana, or nut base. Check out some of the best here: http://www.buzzfeed.com/rachelysanders/amazing-vegan-ice-cream-recipes

—

LINDA'S FAV CHOCOLATE ICE CREAM (GLUTEN FREE, DAIRY FREE)

INGREDIENTS

1 3/4 cups (1 can) full fat coconut milk (organic when possible)
1 cup unsweetened vanilla almond milk
2 tablespoons ground chia seeds (grind in coffee grind to fine powder)
2/3 cup unsweetened cocoa powder (preferably raw organic)
1 teaspoon pure vanilla extract
1/4 cup + 2 Tbsp raw sugar ground in a coffee grinder (may use honey)

INSTRUCTIONS

Place coconut and almond milk, ground chia, cocoa powder, vanilla and sugar in a blender and blend well. Transfer to a mixing bowl, cover and refrigerate until chilled through - at least a couple hours.

Once chilled, pour into pre-chilled ice cream maker and follow the maker's directions. (Or, pour into a freezer-safe container, cover and freezer, taking out to stir every couple hours to aerate.)

Once the ice cream is at soft-peak stage if you are hand stirring, or at the end of the ice cream maker's churning process, stir in any extras you like such as chopped nuts, crystalized ginger chunks, cherries or strawberries, etc. Then spoon into a freezer storage container. Smooth the top with a spoon, cover and freeze until hard. Or, if you let your family taste it, there won't be any left to freeze.

Restart your exercise:

Is it too cold or too hot to go for a walk outside? Do you have stairs in your house? This is a perfect day to do your Intensity training.

Run up the stairs, walk back down, then breathe for 30 seconds. Now do it again. Repeat 7 more times. Increase the breathing time between if you need to so that your heart rate slows slightly between each set.

No stairs? Try planking. It requires nothing but some floor space and sheer will power. It will tone up your core and tighten your abs. A beginner usually can't do more than 3 minutes and that is including rest periods. So go slow and work up until you can do 12 minutes. There are plenty of free demos on the internet to see what a 12-minute routine would be.

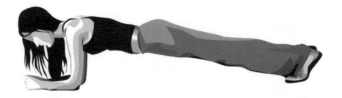

Correct form

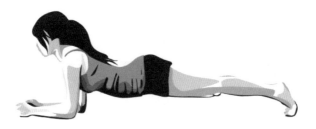

Incorrect form

Release the toxins:

Today's no-no relates to sunscreen. Used winter and summer, sunscreen creates a lot of controversy. One side says to use it all the time to avoid cancer while the other side says avoid it all the time because it causes cancer as well as vitamin D deficiency. So what is the truth? Personally, I side with the "it causes cancer" group if you are talking about commercial big-brand sunscreens loaded with chemicals. There are good organic oil types that are very safe to use, but even those will cause vitamin D issues so should be used judiciously and allow for some sun time. Did you know that natural food-based parabens offer a natural good sun burn protection? The synthetic parabens are cancer causing so avoid anything that is laboratory created parabens. There is a world of difference in food-based parabens that feed the body. There is lots of research to show damage from commercial chemical sunscreens and very little to show that using it prevents skin cancer. So what are the main culprits in commercial sunscreen and other body products?

According to the Environmental Working Group, watch out for this:

OXYBENZONE

Commonly used in sunscreens, the chemical oxybenzone penetrates the skin, gets into the bloodstream and acts like estrogen in the body. It can trigger allergic reactions. Data are preliminary, but studies have found a link between higher concentrations of oxybenzone and health harms. One study has linked oxybenzone to endometriosis in older women; another found that women with higher levels of oxybenzone during pregnancy had lower birth weight daughters.

More than 40 percent of all beach and sport sunscreens contain oxybenzone. And this:

RETINYL PALMITATE, OR SYNTHETIC VITAMIN A

The sunscreen industry adds a form of vitamin A to 12 percent of SPF moisturizers and 20 percent of beach and sport sunscreens. Retinyl palmitate is an antioxidant that slows skin aging, but studies by federal government scientists indicate that it may speed the development of skin tumors and lesions when on skin in the presence of sunlight. EWG recommends that consumers avoid sunscreens, lip products and skin lotions that contain vitamin A, also listed as retinyl palmitate, retinyl acetate or retinol.

Avoid the garbage in commercial sunscreen, but be wise. Find a good quality organic sunscreen, cover up, stay out of the sun at peak periods, and get your food based-parabens that the body uses efficiently when packaged along with the fiber and enzymes that occur naturally within the whole food source. (Commonly found in various vegetable foods, such as barley, strawberries, black currants, peaches, carrots, onions, cocoa-beans, and vanilla beans).

—

DAY 27

The wonderful thing to understand is that the energy that you radiate or send out attracts other situations, events, persons, etc. which are in harmony with your internal energy field.

~ DistantHealing.com

Retrain your thoughts:

Did you get that? You attract to you that which you radiate out. So if you are feeling miserable and grumpy, that is what you will find. If you are feeling joy and peace, that is what you will find. It is as Wayne Dyer tells in his story: When a fellow considered moving to Florida, he visited the neighborhood where they thought they'd like to live. He asked a few people how their neighbors were. One guy said that it wasn't very friendly and he didn't like it. But another said it was wonderful and they had great friends and neighbors all over the neighborhood. He asked each one about where they came from and how their neighbors were there. Wouldn't you know, each one got exactly what they expected and felt it would be like.

If you want to change your situation, your relationship, or your job, then change yourself first and the rest will follow. Deal with what makes you worry. Root out the root of bitterness and anger. Clear the doubt and fear. Make room for a new vibe and that is what you will get.

Reduce your stress:

Never be afraid to admit that you need a little help dealing with your stress. We all have our own blind spots. We all create our own defense shields that hide the bad side from us. Someone who is less attached to the outcome, who can view you from a more neutral position, can see what you can't. Seek out a natural practitioner to help you.

Redefine your diet:

Love your creamy soups and sauces? There are ways to achieve the same with much healthier ingredients. This is my take on it.

—

CREAMY SAUCE

2 tablespoons olive oil
2 medium shallots, diced
8 large cloves garlic, minced/grated
Sea salt and black pepper
3–4 tablespoons chickpea flour, or organic corn starch, or tapioca powder

2.5 cups unsweetened almond milk (make your own or use a plain organic one)

In a large frying pan over medium-low heat, add 2 tbsp olive oil and the garlic and shallot. Add a pinch of salt and black pepper and stir frequently, cooking for 3–4 minutes until softened and fragrant.

Stir in 3–4 tbsp thickener of choice and mix with a whisk. Once combined, slowly whisk in the almond milk a little at a time so clumps don't form. Add another healthy pinch of salt and black pepper, bring to a simmer and continue cooking for another 4–5 minutes to thicken. Taste and adjust seasonings as needed.

If you want an extra-creamy sauce, use an immersion blender to blend the sauce until creamy and smooth. Simmer on low heat until thickened.

Use on pasta, spaghetti squash, or on the top of lasagna instead of cheese. Be creative. I like to throw in a dash of Worcestershire sauce and some oregano when I serve it on spaghetti squash.

Restart your exercise:

What are you doing today? Walk, Tibetan 5, Yoga? Just do something. No excuses.

Release the toxins:

BPA stands for bisphenol A, which is an industrial chemical used to make two common synthetics. One is polycarbonate, which is a shatterproof plastic used to make many products including drink and food containers as well as dental fillings, eyeglass lenses, DVDs, CDs, electronics and sports equipment. BPA is also used to make epoxy resins, which are used in industrial adhesives and coatings which line most of the 131 billion food and beverage cans made in the U.S. annually. (Environmental Working Group)

Bisphenol A is an endocrine disruptor, meaning that it interferes with production, secretion, transport, action, function and/or elimination of natural hormones. BPA imitates our body's own hormones in a way that has been documented to be very detrimental for our health. Endocrine disruptors falsely tell the body's cells that the hormone estrogen is around, causing all sorts of troubling developmental and reproductive consequences.

BPA is known to be particularly dangerous for pregnant women, infants and children. Some effects of BPA have been linked to reproductive disorders, male impotence, heart disease, type 2 diabetes, brain function, memory and learning, breast cancer and asthma to name a few. Canada has banned BPA in baby bottles, but somehow declares it safe for other food containers.

Is BPA-free safe? They have to substitute BPA with something, right? Products that are BPA-free are simply made with bisphenol-S, or BPS. BPS is less known but it shares a similar structure and versatility to BPA and has similar hormone-mimicking characteristics to BPA. BPA and BPS are not the only ingredients in plastic – there are a laundry list of chemicals that make up these containers. There is bisphenol AF and AB, bisphenol B and BP, bisphenol C, E, F, G, M, S and others!

You can't avoid chemicals. They're in our air, water and food. We are surrounded by chemicals and pollution on a daily basis. Fortunately, there are a few things you can do to reduce the amount of nasty chemicals from plastics in your life.

1.   Choose glass for water bottles, glasses, mugs, and pitchers. Watch out for metal

bottles that have a BPA/S liner sprayed inside.

2. Throw out plastic food containers. Use glass or stainless steel instead.

3. If you insist on reheating things in the microwave, don't do it in plastic. Switch the food to a ceramic or glass container to heat up, or better yet, do it on the stove or a toaster oven.

4. Learn to can and preserve your own food in glass jars. Yes, it takes time but it is so worth the effort. Otherwise, eat fresh or frozen. Avoid commercially canned foods.

—

DAY 28

If you were brainwashed into believing that it's 'really hard' to make it in (insert whatever you think is really hard) ... that you need to struggle and be happy just getting by...my advice is to do everything within your power to CLEANSE yourself of this mentality before doing anything else.

~ Kevin Doherty

Retrain your thoughts:

When you believe something is really hard, you make it become that way. You miss the details or alternate routes that would simplify it because you aren't looking for them. If you believe it is really hard to make money, you will accept jobs that take a lot of effort and set yourself up for a lot of work. What if you changed your belief into that it is easy to make money. You might have the same job but your mindset will help you find the efficiencies, changes, and routines that can make a big difference.

Who says you need to struggle and just get by? Where did that belief come from and why do you hang on to it? What could your life be like if you didn't believe that?

Living in the now, accepting that what is, just is, ceasing the struggle and letting go of a required outcome can have a huge impact on how your daily life plays out.

Reduce your stress:

Do the Belief System Elimination on the thought above. Do both the positive and the negative:

- ✓ It is really hard to (insert your thought).

- ✓ It is easy to (insert your thought).

- ✓ I need to struggle and just get by.

- ✓ I don't need to struggle and just get by.

Redefine your diet:

Butter is good for you, especially organic butter. You may be dairy-free, but butter doesn't really count because it is a good fat that your body uses. The problem with butter is that it is usually slathered on a bagel, toast, muffin, or bun. The carbs and sugars in the bread product cause the body to gain weight and increase the bad LDL. The butter doesn't make you fat – it's what you put it on that does. Put your butter on vegetables. Be

Mongolian and melt it into your tea (careful, as hot fats burn more than hot liquids). Most of what you have been told about fat and cholesterol we now know is wrong. Fat doesn't make you fat. Your body requires fats to mineralize teeth and absorb many minerals. It also uses it as energy.

Restart your exercise:

Try a different time of day. See if a walk after dinner refreshes you and gives you more energy to do things in the evening. If you haven't tried it yet, see if doing something first thing in the morning works for you. Some people actually find they like it and it gives them a boost for the day. Drink water before, and eat protein afterwards-avoid the carbohydrate laden post-workout snacks.

Release the toxins:

PERFLUORINATED CHEMICALS (PFCS)

The perfluorinated chemicals used to make non-stick cookware can stick to *you*. Careful of stain-resistant clothing and carpets too. And don't forget, they are in the lining of microwave popcorn bags and your Gore-Tex shoes and raincoat. These chemicals have been proven toxic and carcinogenic in animals. Perfluorochemicals are so widespread and extraordinarily persistent that 99 percent of Americans have these chemicals in their bodies. One particularly notorious compound called PFOA has been shown to be "completely resistant to biodegradation." In other words, PFOA doesn't break down in the environment – ever. That means that even if the chemical was banned after decades of use, it would be showing up in people's bodies for countless generations to come. This is worrisome, since PFOA exposure has been linked to decreased sperm quality, low birth weight, kidney disease, thyroid disease and high cholesterol, among other health issues. Scientists are still figuring out how PFOA affects the human body, but animal studies have found that it can affect thyroid and sex hormone levels.

To avoid it, skip non-stick pans as well as stain and water-resistant coatings on clothing, furniture, carpets, and food packaging. You can safely use ceramic coating on pans. It also appears that silicone coating on pans is safe unless used at over 400 degrees F.

Week 5:
I become who I believe I am

Life has no Remote so get up and change it yourself.

~ Unknown

You have made it past the magic 21 days needed to create new habits. How are you feeling?

Now it is not about a plan or a diet, it is becoming a way of life. These last three days will just cement that way into a familiar pattern.

You have seen by now that you have control over how you react. You can take control over your environment. You can change the way your body responds to stress. You can organize your schedule and do what is important to you. Your new way of life is established. It is up to you to keep it.

There are just a few topics left to tackle: the good and the bad about fat, rest, and sleep.

DAY 29

A knight in shining armour is a man who has never had his metal truly tested.

~ Unknown

Retrain your thoughts:

There will be falls and hard days. There will be times that work or emergencies or holidays and special events will prevent you from following your new lifestyle. So, accept it. That's life. Do what you need to do, or enjoy a few days of indulgence, and then polish up your armor, repair any damage, get back on your horse and carry on. A lifestyle isn't about what any one day looks like – it is made up of the day-after-day habit. It is what is normal for you. Don't judge your lifestyle by any given day.

Reduce your stress:

Rest is a key to reducing stress. Most of us don't even know what rest means. Many people think it means not working or sleeping. Wrong. Rest is the state of relaxed calm in the physical body, while the mind is still and quiet. The brain actually needs an off period when it isn't thinking in order to run its own cleaning cycle. When your brain never stops, it doesn't have the opportunity to clean the toxins and rebuild. You need rest. Sleep is not rest. During sleep your brain is actually very active running cleaning cycles for the rest of the body and dreaming to process all the emotional content of the day.

So rest is lying or sitting still and shutting off the thinking. Let the brain be still. No, it is not impossible. It just takes some training and practice.

Here are some hints on how to start. Your goal is to get up to about 15 minutes a day as a minimum.

Find a quiet place. Be still and let your body relax. Now whenever a thought drifts into your awareness, tell it to go away. If you need to, write it down so you won't forget it. Just keep telling your thoughts, not now. If you need to, gently observe your breathing. Just notice it. Don't control it or count it, just let your attention rest on it.

If you are not used to resting, one minute can seem like a long time. Keep at it and build it up to 15 minutes. If you fall asleep it means you aren't getting enough sleep. Often once you have learned how to rest, you will find you need less sleep. If you use music, it must be instrumental only – no words to distract the attention of the mind. It should be 60 beats per min, which is the resting heart rate.

Redefine your diet:

You've probably heard that "fat makes you fat," and you actually believed it. But truth be told, being fat has nothing to do with the amount of fat you consume.

OK, from a simple caloric standpoint, this misconstrued statement may somehow make sense. In fact, a gram of fat has nine calories, whereas a gram of proteins and carbohydrates each contain four calories. Now, even though calories contribute to weight conditions, they are just an itty-bitty part of the whole story.

To clear up this popular calorie myth, here's exactly what happens when you consume calories:

See, a calorie isn't just a calorie. What your body does with the calorie you consume is what actually counts. And, like we all know, calories are what generate the energy that our body needs for normal functioning. From this statement, it's clear that fats have a higher calorie count, but the calories you take from eating fats will never be more than what your body needs.

Let's pick a carrot, for example. Once you're done eating that one carrot – which of course has a lower calorie count – you'd have enjoyed your snack and that's the end of it; no more carrots, unless you have a thing for carrots. The same illustration can also be used on fats.

On the flip side, try picking a potato chip. Once you've finishing snacking on that single serving of potato chips, you'll probably not be satisfied until you've cleared out the whole bag, which is a number of servings. Far worse, your satisfied salt fix would in turn start yearning for something sugary to balance it out. And before you know it, you'll be stuffing your body with that one thing that should be avoided at all cost – sugar.

What's even scarier about sugar and starchy carbohydrates is the chemical substance stuffed in them – the excitotoxin. For your information, this is the chemical substance that usually blows your appetite, making it impossible for you to survive on a single serving of sugary products.

Although the fats we consume share a name with the fat that's responsible for our big bellies and chunky thighs, it categorically doesn't spur the hormonal dance that's responsible for the formation of this internal fat. What triggers the creation of such fats is either the sugar or the starchy carbohydrates we consume and the emotional stress that triggers the craving in the first place.

Here's a clear picture of what usually happens…

Every time you eat anything sweet, your blood sugar level rises quickly, triggering your pancreas to secrete insulin, the hormone responsible for getting rid of excess sugar from your blood. Now instead of carrying this sugar away into, say, your urinary tract or somewhere else where it would never become a problem, this insulin usually converts the excess sugar into fats before storing it in our bellies and thighs. To be clear, it starts by storing the sugar as glycogen, and once the glycogen stores are full, it stores it as triglycerides – or fat, in layman's language.

Besides stimulating the production of insulin, sugar also prevents glucagon from being operational in your body. Sorry for being a little technical here, but it's helpful for you to know. Glucagon is the hormone that mobilizes the stored sugar back into your bloodstream for energy use. These two hormones are never present in the bloodstream at the same time. In simple words, if insulin in activated, glucagon will definitely not be there to stop it from using the excess sugar in your bloodstream to create the lumpy thighs and the chubby belly you dislike.

Fat doesn't mobilize insulin…

Instead of helping sugar to stimulate the release of insulin, what fat does is slow down your sugar spike, thus reducing the sugar surge and mitigating some of the ill-fated effects of sugar. That said, anyone who advises you to go for a fat-free dessert is literally advising you to let the excess sugar in your bloodstream make you fat.

Fats make your stomach full…

Unlike sugar, fats reduce your appetite. Their digestion triggers your satiation mechanism, thus reducing your hunger pangs. In fact, it's for this reason that anyone who ever suggested a low-fat diet to you actually directed you down the wrong road. The truth is that your body needs fats to stay satisfied, despite the number of calories you take.

For sugars, or foods that quickly convert to sugar in your bloodstream (starchy or processed carbs like cereals, pastas, bread or potatoes), there's no satisfied feeling once eaten. That's to say they will be inspiring an overeating binge the moment you eat them. Actually, when the insulin has fully converted all the sugars in your bloodstream into the disdained belly and thigh fat, you'll instantly start craving more sugar. And by getting more, you'll be making fat storage a continuous process, thus gaining more and more weight as days go by.

So no matter what the medical field and the food marketer tells you, biology says avoid sugars and processed foods. Eat good quality fats like avocados, nuts and seeds, fish, coconut oil, and olives. Avoid sugars and processed foods and your body will begin to lose the fat you don't want.

Restart your exercise:

You are on your own now. You know the drill. Lay out your plan for the week and go do it.

Release the toxins:

We have just a few more chemicals in the "plastics" range. These ones are **glycol ethers.**

Shrunken testicles: do I have your full attention yet? This is one thing that can happen to rats exposed to chemicals called glycol ethers, which are common solvents in paints, cleaning products, brake fluid and cosmetics. Worried? You should be. The European Union says that some of these chemicals "may damage fertility or the unborn child." Studies of painters have linked exposure to certain glycol ethers to blood abnormalities and lower sperm counts. And children who were exposed to glycol ethers from paint in their bedrooms had substantially more asthma and allergies.

Check out Environmental Working Group's Guide to Healthy Cleaning (www.ewg.org/guides/cleaners/) and avoid products with ingredients such as **2-butoxyethanol (EGBE) and methoxydiglycol (DEGME)**.

When you have your house painted, be sure to choose non-VOC paint and leave the windows open for a few days before you sleep in the room.

DAY 30

Two things to remember in life: Take care of your thoughts when you are alone and take care of your words when you are with people.

~ Unknown

Retrain your thoughts:

I love this thought because it forces me to deal with my stress, self-sabotage, and subconscious drivers. Of course using the tools in the "Reduce your stress" section is a huge part of taking care of my thoughts when I am alone. Knowing that I am doing what is right for me, following the path that leads to long-term success as I define it for my life and being rock solid in my commitment to taking care of myself in the midst of a life dedicated to helping others, allows me to take care of my words with others. I don't have to defend myself, or excuse or explain myself. I don't have to preach or push others, I just do what I need to do, let my actions lead by example and set a path for others to follow. When they are ready, they will come along and then it is time to talk. For today, I just need to be true to myself and express love and concern with no judgment, letting others deal with their own stuff. When others attack or belittle or complain about my diet or my schedule or my whatever, I don't have to respond. I just have to accept that what is right for me is not for everyone and if they have a problem with it, it is their problem, not mine. My goal is to be at peace with all.

Reduce your stress:

Make a plan for the next two weeks – that's right, not just the next two days. Lay out your next two weeks of what you will do to control and release stress. Use breathing techniques, relaxation techniques, tapping, ESR (Emotional Stress Relief), BSE (Belief System Elimination), visualization, rest, sleep and anything else you may know. Just make a plan for something every day and stick to it.

Redefine your diet:

You do need fats. But, there are good fats and not good fats, and it is not what you have been told by food marketers or even doctors. For the past 30 years they have vilified saturated fats such as eggs, butter, coconut oil and nuts. We now know that the research that identified coconut as bad for you was done for economic purposes by the seed oil marketers to promote soy, corn, and canola oils instead. Turns out that the health damage is from the soy, corn, and canola, rather than from the coconut. Refined seed oils, particularly canola, are an omega 6 fat that is inflammatory by nature, and those three sources of oil are almost all genetically modified with a toxin. Avoid soy oil, corn oil, and canola oil like the plague.

We also now know that the fats in eggs and butter do not contribute to heart disease. People ate eggs for breakfast for centuries without increased heart disease. It was when the emphasis was put onto cereals, breads, and grains for breakfast that heart disease started to skyrocket. However, instead of pushing back on the grains, they cut out the eggs. When marketers do the research, they can make it say whatever they want. The truth is irrelevant.

Now that is not to say all eggs and meat are just fine. They are not. Given the factory farm and the contamination of the animals' food sources, and the "supplements" they are given so that they don't die when crammed into confined quarters and fed unnatural foods, the eggs and beef are contaminated and should not be eaten. However, organic, grass-fed, free-range, carefully cared for local small farm products are superior on every index and will nourish your health and provide the fats you need.

Avoid liquid seed oils, particularly canola and soy or corn oils that are genetically modified.

Avoid oils that are cooked into processed foods and prepared meals that contain lots of sugar and carbs.

Use coconut oil, avocados, nuts, whole-grain flax, and organic free-range eggs.

Restart your exercise:

Follow your plan.

Release the toxins:

Three plastics have been shown to leach toxic chemicals when heated, worn or put under pressure. Yesterday we looked at polycarbonate, which leaches **bisphenol A**. Tomorrow we will look at polystyrene, better known as Styrofoam, which leaches **styrene**. Today's focused no-no is PVC, or polyvinyl chloride, which breaks down into **vinyl chloride** and usually contains phthalates that can leach in heat.

Your shower curtain may be killing you. Vinyl chloride is formed in the manufacture of polyvinyl chloride (PVC) or Number 3 plastic. It was one of the first chemicals designated as a known human carcinogen by the National Toxicology Program (NTP) and the International Agency for Research on Cancer (IARC). It has also been linked to increased mortality from breast cancer among workers involved in its manufacture.

Most cheap shower curtains are made from PVC. Every time you stand in that hot shower and enjoy that hot relaxing steam, you are breathing in carcinogenic chemicals. The heat releases the dangerous chemicals from the vinyl and you breathe it in. Change your shower curtain to a rubber or cloth one.

So if all this has you freaked out about plastics, check around and see what else is made of plastic and what the plastics contain. They are not all the same. Here is a Hyperlink http://io9.com/how-to-recognize-the-plastics-that-are-hazardous-to-you-461587850

with a great article that lays out the seven types of plastic, each with their little triangle and number that tells you what is what. Number 2 and Number 5 are considered "safe" but should not be heated, such as in a microwave, left in a hot car, left sitting in the sun, etc. Learn to look for the little triangle and number. Simply don't buy things that come in plastics other than Number 2 and Number 5, and even with those be careful.

—

DAY 31

The key to the ability to change is a changeless sense of who you are, what you are about and what you value.

~ Stephen Covey

Retrain your thoughts:

You have been through a lot of change this month, but you have deepened your own sense of self, and your ability to center and ground yourself. You have developed a foundation from which you can make choices and changes based on who you are and what is right for you. You will face many more changes in life but you don't need to feel buffeted around by the howling storm. The waves may crash around you but when you know who you are and how to keep yourself tethered to your core values and purposes, those storms make you stronger. Great old trees don't get to be strong and grounded by living in perfect weather. They get to be strong by withstanding the onslaught of the annual storms and seasons and growing roots to strengthen the systems in the face of threat. They seem hard and solid but they are actually quite flexible and move with the wind. Their roots grow and develop to offset the winds above.

The trunk is strong and moves within a range of its core but the further out the branches and the leaves, the more flexible they are. Your changeless identity will anchor you while the leaves will come and go with the seasons and the storms. So much of what we try to hold on to are just the leaves. Let them go. New and better ones will grow back.

Reduce your stress:

Make a plan for the following two weeks – you did two weeks yesterday, so two weeks more now will give you month planned out. What you will do to control and release stress? Use breathing techniques, relaxation techniques, tapping, ESR (Emotional Stress Relief), BSE (Belief System Elimination), visualization, rest, sleep and anything else you may know. Just make a plan for something every day and stick to it.

Redefine your diet:

We are still on the topic of fats. There is one more type of fat that we need to discuss: Trans-fat. Whenever you see the words "partially hydrogenated oils"…put it down and walk away.

Trans-fats are unsaturated fats which are rarely present in nature but are created artificially in a lab. Trans-fat is made when a liquid vegetable oil is changed into a solid fat. Trans-fat is often added to processed foods because it can improve taste and texture and helps the food stay "fresh" longer. Although trans-fats are edible, consumption of them is known to increase the risk of coronary heart disease in part by raising levels of the lipoprotein LDL (so-called "bad cholesterol"), lowering levels of the lipoprotein HDL ("good cholesterol"), and increasing triglycerides in the bloodstream, thereby promoting inflammation throughout the body.

Read the labels. Beware of products that say "0 Trans-fat" on the nutrition label. Just because the Nutrition Facts label says the product has "0 g Trans-fat," that doesn't necessarily mean it has no trans-fats. By an FDA sleight of hand, it could have up to half a gram of trans-fats per serving. Look at the actual ingredients. If it says "hydrogenated" or "partially hydrogenated," don't buy it and don't eat it.

Restart your exercise:

You have a plan, stick to it.

Release the toxins:

Polystyrene (PS) Sometimes called Styrofoam, this is a plastic that's commonly found in food service items like cups, plates, bowls, cutlery, hinged take out containers (clamshells), meat and poultry trays, rigid food containers (e.g. yogurt), and aspirin bottles. Polystyrene is also used to make protective foam packaging for furniture.

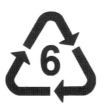

This is another plastic you'll want to avoid. A fundamental problem is that **styrene** can leach from polystyrene. Styrene has been linked to cancer, but the Environmental Protection Agency has not given it a formal carcinogen classification. That said, the EPA admits there's an association to an increased risk of leukemia and lymphoma (among other things). Other studies show that styrene can act as a neurotoxin in the long term. Studies on animals report harmful effects of styrene on red blood cells, the liver, kidney, and stomach organs. The NIHL lists styrene as a probable carcinogen, but says that the styrene leached from polystyrene food containers is at "very low" levels. It also notes that styrene is known to cause lung tumors in mice.

A 2007 study showed that, in Styrofoam and PS cups, "Hot water was found to be contaminated with styrene and other aromatic compounds." Temperature was shown to play a major role in the leaching of styrene, but whether or not styrene leaches into food and water at lower temperatures from polystyrene is a claim that is still contested. Still, as the 2007 study concludes, "Considering the toxic characteristic of styrene and leaching in water and other products, PS material should be avoided for food packaging."

Did you know that one of the highest sources of human contamination with polystyrene comes from cigarettes? Even second-hand smoke contains the released styrene. So…no smoking.

You can also read the CDC's official statement on styrene here (http://www.atsdr.cdc.gov/toxfaqs/tf.asp?id=420&tid=74). And Health Canada's is here (http://www.ec.gc.ca/ese-ees/default.asp?lang=En&n=35DA297C-1).

THE FIRST DAY OF THE REST OF YOUR LIFE.

You made it! I trust you have visible results from all your physical workouts and clean-ups, and invisible, but just as true, results in your heart and mind where you have let go of stress and gained control over some of the sub-conscious thoughts that kept you stuck until now.

With these major strands in place in your life and habits firmly established you will be able to move forward with confidence and peace. If you ever feel yourself slipping back into old patterns, just do the 30 days again. As you educate your family and move them onto a healthier track in life too, it will reinforce your own patterns. The beauty is you can teach your children these skills and habits early in life so that they will have a foundation from which to handle the stresses they face. I teach the ESR to children as young as 6 years old to help them handle stress in school.

I would love to hear your experiences, successes and challenges, and the results you get from following the plan. Please post your comments on my Facebook www.facebook.com/easthousehealth or submit feedback via my webpage www.easthousecentre.com

Here's to your new lifestyle!

APPENDIX A:
Core Beliefs and Life Issues

Listen to your own self-talk

Use these modals – am, can, could, do, might, must, need, ought, shall, should, want, would and their negative counterparts

Use these adverbs – always, constantly, continuously, never

Health	Feeling incompetent (not good enough)
I never sleep well	I am useless
I always have to get up in the night	I am not good enough
I can't heal myself	I will never achieve anything
	I am awkward

Self-Worth	Feeling unlovable (not good enough)
I am untalented, unintelligent and unattractive	Nobody cares about me
I am stupid	I don't deserve to be loved
I am ugly	There must be something wrong with me
I will never amount to anything People always walk all over me	I do not love myself
	I don't deserve happiness
Self-Respect	**Feeling unwanted**
I am not worthy of respect	Nobody wants to spend time with me
Other people take me for granted	I don't matter
My parents didn't respect me	Nobody listens to me
My sisters take advantage of me	I am a burden
	I am a pest

Security	Feeling different
It is not safe to be out at night alone	Other people are more important than I am
I never feel safe in multi-story parkades	I don't fit in (anywhere)
The world is not a safe place	I am always left out
Authority is scary	Wherever I am, I am unwelcome
	I'm nothing
	I stick out like a sore thumb
	I can never be myself
	I can't cope with criticism Everyone thinks I am stupid
Success	**Feeling useless**
Nothing ever goes right for me	I am useless (at ....)
Money is difficult to come by honestly	I will never be any good at (.......................)
I can't afford to take time off	I never start what I finish
Life is a continuous struggle	I am so disorganized
My boss never sees me	

Control

Pleasing other people is the right thing to do

Being there for others keeps them happy

My finances are always out of control

Feeling hopeless

I'll never amount to much

I can't handle change

No matter how hard I try I can never get it right

I can never make decisions

I never stick with any decisions I make

I am hopeless
(at.......................)

Feeling powerless

I am weak

I can't stand up for myself

I don't dare stand up for myself

I am powerless to change

I always leave myself open to abuse/being used

I must obey other people's dictates

Forgiving other people is hard

I can't get in touch with my emotions

Feeling insecure

Life is hard

Men (Women) take advantage of me
Nobody respects me

People cannot be trusted
People are not reliable

You can't trust ....
(men, women, alcoholics)

It is dangerous to allow other people to get close

© Ann Parker – Health Kinesiology NZ 2011

BELIEF SYSTEM ELIMINATION
DEVELOPED BY JIMMY SCOTT, PH.D.

This BS Elimination procedure works very quickly to eliminate or reduce beliefs that are deeply held and are holding us back, keeping us in emotional captivity.

Negative statements we hear, especially if spoken by people we trust or who "have power over us" (parents, teachers, authorities, etc), can become locked into the bioenergy system, and held as true, long after the initial statement or situation was consciously forgotten. These beliefs help shape our behaviour and attitudes toward ourselves and the world.

Examples:

- I never finish what I start.

- I'll always be hopeless at maths.

- I'll never amount to much.

- I'm lazy/stupid/untidy/disorganized/hopeless. etc. etc.

- People are not reliable.

- You cannot trust a woman.

- Alcoholics are scum.

- Black people are violent.

- Homosexuals are immoral.

- Everybody loves me.

- I love everybody.

- I can't do mathematics.

- I can't cook.

Verbally identify the belief system to be eliminated. Key words include: 'I never...', 'I always....', 'I can't...', 'I shouldn't...', 'I should'..., 'It's impossible...' etc. However, either negative or positive words can occur in the items.

Speak the phrase deliberately and at a normal pace. **Typically it only takes 15 to 30 seconds to complete an item.** Sometimes it can take a minute or more. Just like in most energy work a deep breath or yawn usually occurs with the energy shift at the completion of the correction. Pinching is done while the statement is repeated out loud until a shift or release is felt.

Specific areas on the head are stimulated, to create changes in the nervous system / bioenergy system. The skin is lightly pinched:

Horizontally on the back of the head at the occiput, on the soft tissue between each inion with finger tips about 2 cm or 3/4 inch apart, and, simultaneously vertically on the midline at the front of the head, with one finger just in the usual hairline and the other just below, about 2 cm or 3/4 inch apart.

APPENDIX B:
Tibetan 5 Exercises

Exercise 1: Stand upright, extend your arms at shoulder level away from your body and spin clockwise (if looking at a clock face on the floor). Keep your eyes looking directly in front of you, do not focus on any one point, let your vision blur as you spin. Turn up to 21 times or until you feel unstable or dizzy. Start where you are comfortable and work your way up to 21 spins. Speed is not so important

> **Breathing:** Breathe in and out of your stomach. When you stop spinning, breath even more deeply from your stomach until your head stops spinning and your balance returns to normal.

Exercise 2: Lay down on your back with your arms to your side, palms up, keep your legs straight, begin your inhalation, raise your legs off the ground until as high as possible and pick your head off the ground, bending your neck with your chin falling toward your chest. Begin your exhalation and return to lying flat on the ground. If you need to, bend your knees to raise the legs until your stomach strengthens. If your feel discomfort, place your hands (palms facing down) under your buttocks to support your lower spine. Work up to repeating up to 21 times.

Breathe In: Raising your legs and head

Breathe Out: Lowering your legs and head

Exercise 3: Kneel with your legs together, arms extended, palms of your hands on the side of your thighs, drop your chin to your chest, begin your inhalation, raise your head and lean back, move your hands to the back of your thighs and let them drop lower and support your weight, crane your head and neck backward, relax your lower spine. Begin your exhalation; start to come forward back to kneeling position with your head back up in the straight position. Use the weight of your head to come forward instead of forcing your chin to your chest with your muscles. When you lean back, avoid craning your neck, simply let it drop with its own weight. Repeat up to 21 times.

Breathe In: Going backward

Breathe Out: Coming forward

Exercise 4: Sit on the floor, legs a little less than shoulder width apart, arms to your sides with hands extended flat on the ground and fingers pointed forward, drop your head toward your chest, begin your inhalation, raise your buttocks off the ground while bending your knees, shift your weight to your arms/hands and legs/feet, continue to raise your buttocks until your trunk and thighs are parallel to the ground, let your head fall back. Begin your exhalation and return to sitting position with your head dropped forward. Repeating up to 21 times.

Breathe In: Raising off the ground

Breathe Out: Returning back to sitting position

Tips and Recommendations: When you begin this exercise, just try to get from the starting to ending postures. It's easier to do it than read about it. If you have a shoulder injury or cannot complete the movement, don't strain yourself. Check out the alternate on Day 21 p.99.

Exercise 5: Get down on the floor on your hands and knees (in push-up position) with hands and legs a little less than shoulder width apart. Begin your inhalation, come up on your toes with weight in your arms, straighten your legs, arch your back, lean your head back, do not let any of your body touch the ground except for your toes and hands (Cobra in Yoga). Begin your exhalation, bend at the waist, bend your knees, push your buttocks up into the air, make an inverted V shape with your legs and arms straight, tuck your chin toward your chest (Downward Dog in Yoga), and try to put your feet flat on the ground. Begin your next inhalation and repeat up to 21 times.

Breathe In: Raising hips up into an ^ shape - downward dog.

Breathe Out: Hips down & head coming up into cobra.

APPENDIX C:
11 most toxic additives in food you eat every day

—

AVOID THESE

Compiled by Linda Orr Easthouse

1. Artificial Sweeteners

Aspartame (E951), more popularly known as NutraSweet and Equal but now being marketed as AminoSweet, is found in foods labeled "diet" or "sugar-free". Aspartame is believed to be carcinogenic and accounts for more reports of adverse reactions than all other foods and food additives combined. Aspartame is not your friend. Aspartame is a neurotoxin and carcinogen. Known to erode intelligence and affect short-term memory, the components of this toxic sweetener may lead to a wide variety of ailments including brain tumor, diseases like lymphoma, diabetes, multiple sclerosis, Parkinson's, Alzheimer's, fibromyalgia, and chronic fatigue, emotional disorders like depression and anxiety attacks, dizziness, headaches, nausea, mental confusion, migraines and seizures. Acesulfame-K, a relatively new artificial sweetener found in baking goods, gum and gelatin, has not been thoroughly tested and has been linked to kidney tumors.

Watch for it in diet or sugar-free sodas, Diet Coke, Coke Zero, Jell-O (and other gelatins), desserts, sugar-free gum, drink mixes, baking goods, tabletop sweeteners, cereal, breath mints, pudding, Kool-Aid, ice tea, chewable vitamins, and toothpaste.

2. High-Fructose Corn Syrup/Agave Nectar

High fructose corn syrup (HFCS) is a highly-refined artificial sweetener which has become the number one source of calories in America. It is found in almost all processed foods. HFCS packs on the pounds faster than any other ingredient, increases your LDL ("bad") cholesterol levels, and contributes to the development of diabetes and tissue damage, among other harmful effects.

It is found in most processed foods, breads, candy, flavored yogurts, salad dressings, canned vegetables, and cereals. It is used in Canada too, but shows up as "glucose-fructose." Manufacturers got savvy that consumers didn't want HFCS, so they just changed the name.

In many "healthy" foods they substitute agave nectar. It is really the same thing and is not healthy. The hard tuberous root of the agave cactus is ground up like the hard corn stalks are, treated with all kinds of chemicals and processed into "nectar." The name is meant to deceive you into thinking you are getting something like maple syrup or the nectar that the bees collect. It is highly processed, often contaminated with mercury and not worthy of the name "natural." Avoid foods that contain these.

3. *Monosodium Glutamate (MSG / E621)*

MSG is an amino acid used as a flavor enhancer in soups, salad dressings, chips, frozen entrees, and many restaurant foods. MSG is known as an excito-toxin, a substance which overexcites cells to the point of damage or death. Studies show that regular consumption of MSG may result in adverse side effects which include depression, disorientation, eye damage, fatigue, head-aches, and obesity. MSG affects the neurological pathways of the brain and disengages the "I'm full" function. which explains the effects of weight gain.

INGREDIENTS THAT ALWAYS CONTAIN MSG

- Autolyzed yeast
- Calcium caseinate
- Gelatin
- Glutamate
- Glutamic acid
- Hydrolyzed protein
- Sodium caseinate
- Textured protein
- Monosodium glutamate
- Yeast extract
- Yeast food
- Yeast nutrient
- Monopotassium glutamate

INGREDIENTS THAT OFTEN CONTAIN MSG

- Flavors and flavorings
- Seasonings
- Natural flavors/flavorings
- Natural pork flavoring

- Natural beef flavoring
- Natural chicken flavoring
- Soy sauce
- Soy protein isolates
- Soy protein
- Bouillon
- Stock
- Broth
- Malt extract
- Malt flavor
- Barley malt
- Anything enzyme modified
- Carrageenan
- Maltodextrin
- Pectin
- Enzymes
- Protease
- Corn starch
- Citric acid
- Powdered milk
- Anything protein fortified
- Anything ultra-pasteurized

Found in: Chinese food (Chinese restaurant syndrome) many snacks, chips, cookies, seasonings, most Campbell's soup products, frozen dinners, lunch meats

4. Common Food Dyes

Studies show that artificial colorings found in soda, fruit juices and salad dressings may contribute to behavioral problems in children and lead to a significant reduction in IQ. Animal studies have linked other food colorings to cancer. Watch out for these ones:

Table 1: Some of the worst Colour additives approved for use in Canada and their alternate names.

Canadian Name	European Name	USA Names	
Allura Red	E129	Food Red 17, FD&C Red 40	Has been proven to cause thyroid cancer and chromo-somal damage in laboratory animals; may also interfere with brain-nerve transmission
Amaranth	E123	C.I. Food Red No. 9, FD&C Red 2	
Brilliant Blue FCF Found in: candy, cereal, soft drinks, sports drinks and pet foods	E133	Food Blue 2, FD&C Blue 1	Banned in Norway, Finland and France. May cause chromosomal damage
Citrus Red No. 2	None	Citrus Red 2, C.I. Solvent Red 80	

Erythrosine Found in: fruit cocktail, maraschino cherries, cherry pie mix, ice cream, candy, bakery products	E127	Food Red 14, FD&C Red 3, Acid Red 51	Banned in 1990 after eight years of debate from use in many foods and cosmetics. This dye continues to be on the market until supplies run out!
Fast Green FCF	E143	Food Green 3, FD&C Green 3, Solid Green FCF	
Indigotine	E132	FD&C Blue 2, Indigo Carmine	
Ponceau SX	E125	Food Red 2, FD&C Red 4, Scarlet GN	

Sunset Yellow FCF packet soups, breadcrumbs, ice cream, canned fish, lemon curd, hot chocolate mix, some jams and jellies and many medications	E110	Orange Yellow S, FD&C Yellow 6	A synthetic coal tar and azo dye used in fermented foods that must be heat-treated.
Tartrazine American cheese, macaroni and cheese, candy and carbonated beverages, lemonade	E102	FD&C Yellow 5	Banned in Norway and Sweden. Increases the number of kidney and adrenal gland tumors in laboratory animals; may cause chromo-somal damage.

https://www.uoguelph.ca/foodsafetynetwork/artificial-colours

5. Sodium Benzoate and Potassium Benzoate

These preservatives are sometimes added to soda to prevent mold from growing, but benzene is a known carcinogen that is also linked with serious thyroid damage. Dangerous levels of benzene can build up when plastic bottles of soda are exposed to heat or when the preservatives are combined with ascorbic acid (vitamin C). Often found in fruit juices, even those marketed as "healthy."

6. Soybean, Canola and Corn Oil

Nearly 80 percent of all soybean crops grown in the U.S. are genetically modified (GMO) compared to 1996, when only 7 percent were GMO soybeans.

According to the International Service for the Acquisition of Agri-Biotech Applications, 97.5 percent of the canola grown in Canada last year was GMO. Genetically modified crops not only pose environmental dangers, there is a growing concern (and mounting scientific evidence) that genetic engineering of food plant seeds may have an unexpected and negative impact on human health.

7. Propylene glycol (alginate) -E405

This food thickener, stabilizer, and emulsifier is derived from alginic acid esterified and combined with propylene glycol. Bear in mind that even though propylene glycol is used as a food additive, it has many industrial uses including automotive antifreezes and airport runway de-icers.

8. Polysorbate 60

Short for polyoxyethylene-(20)- sorbitan monostearate this emulsifier is widely used in the food industry. Made of made of corn, palm oil and petroleum, this gooey mix can't spoil, so it often replaces dairy products in baked goods and other liquid products.

9. Sodium Nitrate/Sodium Nitrite

Sodium nitrate (or sodium nitrite) is used as a preservative, coloring and flavoring in bacon, ham, hot dogs, luncheon meats, corned beef, smoked fish and other processed meats. This ingredient, which sounds harmless, is actually highly carcinogenic once it enters the human digestive system. There, it forms a variety of nitrosamine compounds that enter the bloodstream and wreak havoc with a number of internal organs, the liver and pancreas in particular. Sodium nitrite is widely regarded as a toxic ingredient, and the USDA actually tried to ban this additive in the 1970s but was vetoed by food manufacturers who complained they had no alternative for preserving packaged meat products. Why does the industry still use it? Simple: this chemical just happens to turn meats bright red. It's actually a color fixer, and it makes old, dead meats appear fresh and vibrant.

Found in: hot dogs, bacon, ham, luncheon meat, cured meats, corned beef, smoked fish or any other type of processed meat.

10. BHA and BHT (E320)

Butylated hydroxyanisole (BHA) and butylated hydrozytoluene (BHT) are preservatives found in cereals, chewing gum, potato chips, and vegetable oils. This common preservative keeps foods from changing color, changing flavor or becoming rancid. It affects the neurological system of the brain, alters behavior and has potential to cause cancer. BHA and BHT are oxidants which form cancer-causing reactive compounds in your body.

Found in: potato chips, gum, cereal, frozen sausages, enriched rice, lard, shortening, candy, Jell-O.

11. Sulfur Dioxide (E220)

Sulfur additives are toxic and in the United States of America, the Federal Drug Administration have prohibited their use on raw fruit and vegetables. Adverse reactions include: bronchial problems particularly in those prone to asthma, hypotension (low blood pressure), flushing tingling sensations or anaphylactic shock. It also destroys vitamins B1 and E. Not recommended for consumption by children. The International Labour Organization says to avoid E220 if you suffer from conjunctivitis, bronchitis, emphysema, bronchial asthma, or cardiovascular disease.

Found in: beer, soft drinks, dried fruit, juices, cordials, wine, vinegar, and potato products.

About the Author

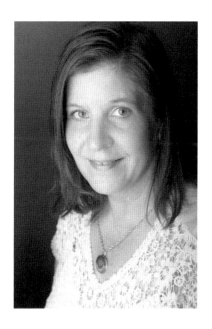

Linda Orr Easthouse has been an internationally certified Health Kinesiology (HK) practitioner for the past ten years, as well as being an HK Instructor and a certified Matrix Energetics practitioner.

Having personally benefited greatly from what she learned in the field, and having helped many others to achieve healthier and happier lifestyles through private healing sessions and her published writing and teaching, as well as the lectures she has given for corporate and non-profit groups on stress management and nutrition as a solution to stress, Easthouse found herself motivated to expand the reach of what she has to offer.

This book is the result.

An organic gardener, Easthouse currently lives in a one-hun-dred-and-three-year-old house in Calgary Alberta, with her husband and youngest son.

For more information about Linda Orr Easthouse:

www.Lindaeasthouse.com

www.easthousecentre.com

www.facebook.com/EasthouseHealth

twitter@easthousecentre

Printed in Canada